MCQ TUTOR: MEDICAL I

MCQ TUTOR:
MEDICAL IMMUNOLOGY

Ruth C. Matthews BSc, MB BS, MSc
*Lecturer in Medical Microbiology and Honorary Senior Registrar,
St Bartholomew's Hospital, London*

and

James P. Burnie MA (Cantab), MRCP, MSc
*Lecturer in Medical Microbiology,
London Hospital, London*

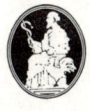

WILLIAM HEINEMANN MEDICAL BOOKS LTD
London

First published 1984
by William Heinemann Medical Books Ltd,
23 Bedford Square,
London WC1B 3HH

ISBN: 0–433–20347–1

Photoset, printed and bound in Great Britain by
Redwood Burn Limited, Trowbridge, Wiltshire

CONTENTS

INTRODUCTION

This book is designed as an examination aid for students of medicine, immunology, medical laboratory sciences and candidates for the primary examinations of the Royal Colleges. It consists of over 300 MCQs which cover both basic and clinical immunology.

The first part of the book distils the basic facts which constitute immunology and presents them as concisely as possible. It offers practice in MCQ questions so that both the facts and their comprehension are tested simultaneously. This is ideal for second MB and for BSc courses in immunology.

As the student progresses to final MB, the second half of the book becomes more useful: MCQs in immunology have now become a feature of the final MB pathology paper. There are clinically orientated chapters which should prove useful in preparing for the papers in medicine.

This book also fills a gap produced by the Royal College of Physicians. The decision to make Part One MRCP more orientated towards basic sciences means that immunology, both basic and clinical, takes on a new importance. As immunology is a rapidly expanding science, there will obviously be increasing scope for such questions. For the Part One MRCP candidate the first half of the book deals with aspects of immunology which are sufficiently non-controversial to be used as material for multiple choice questions. The second half covers the clinical applications of these facts.

In summary, chapters 1 to 7 and 19 will be particularly useful for those studying for the Second MB and Final MB and for those undertaking BSc courses. Chapters 8 to 19 cover areas of the MRCP Part One. The questions should be attempted in the order in which they appear in each chapter, otherwise information contained in a later question may provide the answer to an earlier one. Each stem in each question is independent and all five stems in each case can be true or false.

A mark should be deducted for each incorrect answer and a good candidate should score about 60%.

An extensive bibliography is provided at the end of the book, giving both general suggestions for further reading, and specific references relating to particular groups of questions.

1. STRUCTURE AND FUNCTION OF IMMUNOGLOBULINS

1.1 Which of the following is/are true concerning immunoglobulins?

A. They are glycoproteins.
B. They are split by pepsin into Fc (fraction crystallisable) and monovalent Fab (fraction antigen binding) fragments.
C. They are immunogenic.
D. They consist of variable and constant regions which are coded for by different chromosomes.
E. They travel towards the anode during the electrophoresis of serum.

1.2 Concerning human IgG, which of the following is/are true?

A. It is the major antibody in the primary antibody response to an antigen.
B. It is the major antibody to neutralise bacterial toxins.
C. It is the major antibody which confers natural passive immunity on the fetus.
D. It is divided into five subclasses.
E. It is the immunoglobulin with the strongest precipitating capacity.

1.3 Concerning human IgG, which of the following is/are true?

A. It has a molecular weight of 50 000 d.
B. It is monovalent.
C. It constitutes 60% of immunoglobulin in the serum.
D. It has a higher rate of synthesis than other immunoglobulins.
E. It has a higher rate of degradation than other immunoglobulins.

Answers overleaf

Structure and Function of Immunoglobulins

1.1 A, C

Immunoglobulins are glycoproteins which migrate towards the cathode during electrophoresis. Papain and not pepsin splits them into the Fc and monovalent Fab fragments. Pepsin works above the sulph-hydryl bond and produces a divalent $F (ab')_2$ fragment and a slightly shorter crystallisable (Fc′) fragment. The variable and constant regions are coded for by the same chromosome. Immunoglobulins are long-chain polypeptides and can thus be immunogenic.

1.2 B, C

IgM predominates in the primary and IgG in the secondary antibody response. IgG readily crosses the placenta to reach the fetus. It enters the extravascular space and precipitates soluble antigens, which makes it the most important immunoglobulin in neutralising bacterial toxins. It has four subclasses (IgG1 to 4) and 70% of IgG is IgG1.

1.3 D

IgG is a monomer with two Fab portions and hence is divalent. Each immunoglobulin molecule is able to interact with two antigenic determinants. It has a molecular weight of 150 000 d and constitutes over 75% of serum immunoglobulin. It has a slower rate of degradation and a higher rate of synthesis than other immunoglobulin classes.

Structure and Function of Immunoglobulins

1.4 Concerning human IgM, which of the following is/are true?

   A. Phylogenetically it precedes IgG.
   B. Compared with IgG it has a relatively high avidity and low affinity.
   C. It is a less efficient agglutinator than IgG.
   D. It fixes complement less readily than IgG via the classical pathway.
   E. It is mainly intravascular.

1.5 Concerning human IgA, which of the following is/are true?

   A. It is present in the serum at a lower concentration than IgM and IgG.
   B. It is the predominant immunoglobulin in external secretions and has an important role in preventing the entry of antigens into the body.
   C. It has two subclasses which are present in equal amounts in both serum and secretions.
   D. Monomeric IgA predominates in the secretions and dimeric IgA in the serum.
   E. It activates the classical complement pathway.

1.6 Which of the following is/are true concerning human IgE?

   A. It is found mainly in the skin, respiratory and gastrointestinal tracts.
   B. It aids in the immunological protection of external mucosal surfaces.
   C. It mediates the degranulation of eosinophils when eosinophil-bound IgE reacts with antigen.
   D. It activates the classical complement pathway.
   E. Serum levels may be increased in atopics and in individuals with parasitic infections.

Answers overleaf

3

1.4 A, B, E

Phylogenetically IgM precedes IgG. It has a pentameric structure whereas IgG is a monomer. IgM is produced earlier in the antibody response than IgG and its affinity for the antigen tends to be lower. However, although the affinity between antigen and antibody at each binding site tends to be lower, the increased number of binding sites in the case of pentameric IgM ensures a high avidity. IgM is also a more efficient agglutinator and fixes complement more readily than IgG because of the bonus effect of multivalence. IgM is too large to cross the placenta or leave the intravascular space.

1.5 B

IgM is present in lower amounts than IgA and IgG is present in higher amounts than IgA in the serum. IgA is the predominant immunoglobulin in external secretions where it blocks antigen entry into the body. IgA subdivides into two subclasses, IgA1 and IgA2. IgA1 predominates in the serum. Serum IgA is mainly monomeric in contrast to the secretory form which is mainly dimeric. IgA activates complement by the alternate pathway.

1.6 A, B, E

IgE is found predominantly in the skin, respiratory and gastrointestinal tracts. It provides a back-up system for secretory IgA in that it mops up antigens which bypass the latter. It activates the alternate complement pathway and eosinophils can kill IgE-coated helminths. Degranulation of IgE-coated mast cells and basophils can mediate atopic reactions and anaphylaxis.

1.7 Which of the following is/are true concerning human IgD?

A. It is the predominant immunoglobulin in the colostrum.
B. It is present on the surface of B lymphocytes in the newborn.
C. It has two disulphide bridges between the two heavy chains of the immunoglobulin.
D. It has a molecular weight of 185 000 d.
E. It mediates Rhesus disease of the newborn.

1.8 Which of the following is/are true concerning antibody?

A. It can be induced by a hapten alone.
B. It recognises the three-dimensional shape of the outer electron cloud of an antigen.
C. Its affinity depends upon the sum of attractive and repulsive forces.
D. Its affinity is the strength of interaction of its binding site with an antigenic determinant.
E. Avidity takes into account the valence of the antibody and antigen.

1.9 Which of the following antibodies or parts of antibodies is/are divalent?

A. IgM antibody.
B. Fc.
C. IgD antibody.
D. Fab.
E. $F(ab')_2$.

1.10 A mouse is injected on two separate occasions with staphylococcal toxoid. Which of the following is/are true concerning the antibody response on the second contact?

A. It is mainly IgM.
B. It is detectable after a longer lag phase.
C. It is produced at a higher titre.
D. It is antigen specific.
E. It is mainly of lower affinity than that of the primary response.

Answers overleaf

5

1.7 B, D

IgD has a molecular weight of 185 000 d and is present on the surface of B lymphocytes in the newborn. IgA is the predominant immunoglobulin in the colostrum. IgG mediates Rhesus disease of the newborn. IgD differs from other human immunoglobulins in having only one disulphide bridge between the two heavy chains.

1.8 B, C, D, E

A hapten is a small molecule capable of binding to antibody but not inducing it (e.g. dinitrophenol). However, when it is bound to a carrier it can evoke antibody. Antibody recognises the three-dimensional conformation of an antigen. It binds to it with an affinity dependent on the sum of attractive and repulsive forces. The former include hydrogen bonding, ionic forces, van de Waal's forces and, in an aqueous environment, hydrophobic forces. The latter arise from interpenetration of electron clouds so that the greater the structural complementarity between antigen and antibody, the lower the repulsive force. Avidity includes the increased binding capacity due to the multivalent nature of most biological antigens and antibody ('bonus of multivalence').

1.9 C, E

Fab and Fc are monovalent. The pepsin fragment F $(ab')_2$ is divalent. IgM has a valency of ten, being a pentamer of divalent immunoglobulin chains. IgD is divalent.

1.10 C, D

The antibody produced during a secondary response is mainly IgG, which is produced more quickly and in greater amounts. This is the basis of conferring immunity by vaccination. This adaptation of the immune response is generally antigen specific (exceptions may be referred to as 'anamnestic reactions'). The affinity of secondary antibody tends to be higher, probably due to antigen-driven preferential selection and stimulation of those lymphocytes bearing high-affinity receptors.

Structure and Function of Immunoglobulins

1.11 Which of the following tests can detect as little as 0.001 mg/ml of antibody?

    A. Immunoelectrophoresis.
    B. Bacterial agglutination.
    C. Enzyme-linked immunoassay (ELISA).
    D. Radioimmunoassay (RIA).
    E. Complement fixation test (CFT).

1.12 Which of the following assays directly measures the primary interaction between antibody and antigen and is/are not dependent on secondary interactions?

    A. Ammonium sulphate precipitation (Farr assay).
    B. Quantitative precipitation assay.
    C. Agglutination.
    D. Fluorescence quenching.
    E. Haemolysis.

1.13 The precipitin curve shown in Fig. 1 was obtained by adding increasing amounts of antigen to a fixed concentration of antiserum. The optical densities of the precipitates (in sodium hydroxide) were determined. The supernatants were assayed for the presence of free antibody or antigen by immunodiffusion. Which of the following is/are true concerning the supernatants?

    A. At (i) there was an excess of antibody.
    B. At (ii) there was a small excess of antibody.
    C. At (iii), the point of maximum precipitation, there was no antigen or antibody.
    D. At (iv) there was a small excess of antigen.
    E. At (v) there was an excess of antigen.

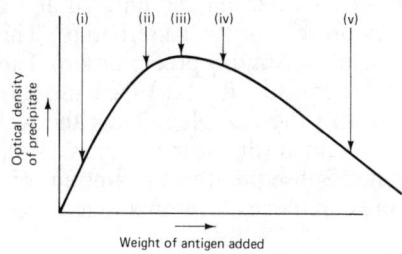

Fig. 1   Precipitin curve   *Answers overleaf*

1.11 C, D

RIA and ELISA are two of the most sensitive assays for measuring antibody. Immunoelectrophoresis is relatively insensitive (minimum detectable 100 mg/ml). The CFT can detect 0.1–1.0 mg/ml. The sensitivity of agglutination tests varies with the assay system being used, but they are less sensitive than RIA or ELISA, e.g. bacterial agglutination with *Salmonella typhi* can detect as little as 0.1 mg/ml antibody.

1.12 A, D

Primary interaction tests depend only on the binding of antibody to antigen and are not dependent upon any secondary manifestations of this event, such as precipitation, agglutination, complement fixation or haemolysis. This is advantageous because such secondary interactions may not occur. These primary binding tests determine the concentration of antibody, by measuring the concentrations of both free and bound antigen after these two have been separated. For example, the Farr assay can be used when the antigen is soluble in 50% saturated ammonium sulphate solution and the antibody is insoluble. An excess of radiolabelled antigen is allowed to react with antibody. Ammonium sulphate is added, precipitating bound antigen–antibody. By comparing the amount of radioactivity in the precipitate with the total radioactivity it is possible to calculate the percentage of antigen bound and therefore the antibody concentration of the serum. Fluorescence quenching is applicable to fluorescent antigens (e.g. fluorescein-labelled drugs), fluorescence being reduced when antibody binds to antigen. Similar assays, by adding an unknown amount of an unlabelled drug to a standard labelled drug with antibody, have been used to measure drug levels.

1.13 A, D, E

The equivalence point occurs when all the antigen and antibody is complexed and neither is present in the supernatant. This occurs at (ii), just before the point of maximum precipitation. The weight of precipitate continues to increase after (ii) because of continued incorporation of antigen into the complex. Thus the weight of the precipitate reaches a maximum at (iii), when there is a small excess of antigen in the supernatant. Subsequently, the amount of precipitate decreases because soluble complexes form in antigen excess.

1.14 At the equivalence point, the optical density (OD) of the precipitate was 0.4 and the weight of the antigen added was 80 µg. Calculate the antibody content of the serum, given that the sample volume was 100 µl and that an OD of 1.0 was given by both 2 mg/ml antigen and 0.695 mg/ml antibody (IgG).

    A. 1.0
    B. 1.25
    C. 2.0
    D. 2.5
    E. 5.0

1.15 Using the same antigen and antibody, the OD of the precipitate in extreme antibody excess was 0.20 per ml in the presence of 10 µg of antigen. Given that the molecular weight of the antibody (IgG) was 150 000 d and that of the antigen 66 420 d, calculate the number of determinants on the antigen.

    A. 12
    B. 6
    C. 3
    D. 2
    E. 1

Answers overleaf

1.14 D

At equivalence, all antigen and antibody is in the precipitate.

$$\text{OD precipitate} = \text{OD antigen} + \text{OD antibody}$$
$$\text{OD precipitate} = 0.40$$

$$\text{OD antigen} = \frac{\text{weight of antigen (mg)}}{\text{weight in mg giving an OD of 1}}$$
$$= \frac{0.08}{2} = 0.04$$

Therefore
$$\text{OD antibody} = 0.40 - 0.04$$
$$= 0.36$$

Therefore
$$\text{amount of antibody} = \frac{(\text{number of mg giving an OD of 1}) \times (\text{OD antibody})}{(\text{sample volume in ml})}$$
$$= \frac{0.695 \times 0.36}{0.1}$$
$$= 2.5 \text{ mg/ml}$$

1.15 B

$$\text{OD of 0.01 mg of antigen} = \frac{1 \times 0.01}{2} = 0.005 \text{ per ml}$$
$$\text{OD of precipitate} = 0.20 \text{ per ml}$$
$$\text{Therefore OD of antibody} = 0.20 - 0.005 = 0.195 \text{ per ml}$$
$$\text{Therefore amount of antibody} = 0.695 \times 0.195 = 0.1355 \text{ mg/ml}$$
$$= 135.5 \text{ µg/ml}$$

At extreme antibody excess, every antigenic determinant is likely to be covered by a separate antibody molecule. So the ratio of the number of molecules of antigen to antibody will give the valency of the antigen:

$$\frac{\text{weight of antigen}}{\text{mol. wt of antigen}} : \frac{\text{weight of antibody}}{\text{mol. wt of antibody}}$$
$$\frac{10}{66\,420} : \frac{135.5}{150\,000} = 0.00015 : 0.000903$$

Therefore the ratio of antibody to antigen molecules is 6.
Therefore, this antiserum recognises 6 determinants on the antigen molecule.

1.16 On the basis of the gell diffusion assay shown in Fig.2, which of the following is/are true concerning antigens X, Y and Z?
HSA, human serum albumin
BSA, bovine serum albumin
anti-HSA, antibody against HSA

A. X is BSA.
B. Y is HSA.
C. Z is HSA.
D. Z is neither HSA nor BSA.
E. Z is BSA and HSA.

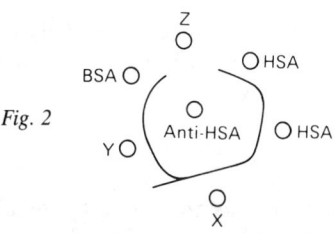

Fig. 2

1.17 In Fig. 3, if X is HSA and Z is transferrin, identify the antiserum W.

A. Anti-BSA only.
B. Anti-HSA only.
C. Anti-transferrin only.
D. Anti-HSA and anti-transferrin.
E. None of these.

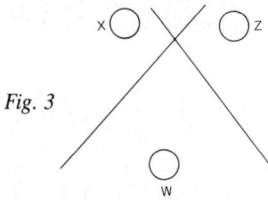

Fig. 3

1.18 Which of the following is/are example(s) of allotypes?

A. λ.
B. IgA2.
C. Oz.
D. Gm
E. Km (Inv).   *Answers overleaf*

11

1.16 D

X is HSA, hence it shows a continuous confluent curve with the HSA (indicating identity) and a spur with Y, which is BSA (indicating partial identity). Y is BSA because it shows a continuous confluent curve with BSA, indicating identity. A spur occurs in reactions of partial identity because the remaining antibody crosses the precipitin line to react with antigen from the adjacent well. Z is neither HSA nor BSA so that it fails to produce a precipitin line with anti-HSA.

1.17 D

W contains anti-HSA and anti-transferrin. This gives two crossing precipitin lines, formed by the antibodies reacting to two unrelated antigens, transferrin and HSA.

1.18 D, E

Allotypic antigenic determinants are coded for by alleles (alternative genes) and are therefore not present in all individuals. They are usually located on the constant part of the immunoglobulin, e.g. the Gm (on IgG) and Am (on IgA) antigens. Isotypes are the different classes, subclasses, types, subtypes and subgroups of immunoglobulins. All these variants are present in any normal individual of a species. They can be detected by innoculation into a different species. Both λ and κ light chains are present in the serum of normal people and therefore these are examples of isotypic variants. The λ chains have amino-acid differences at numbers 190 and 152, the Oz and Kern markers. These are isotypic. In contrast, the κ light chain has an allotypic marker called the Km (Inv) marker.

1.19. Concerning idiotypes, which of the following is/are true?

A. They are located in the constant region of the heavy chain.
B. They are all present together in the serum of any normal individual in a species.
C. They are defined by antisera induced by innoculating antibody into a different species.
D. They can be coded for by germ-line genes.
E. They are thought to be involved in the control of the humoral response.

1.20 Clinically healthy individuals living in the Tropics are likely to differ from healthy Europeans in having which of the following?

A. A higher serum IgM.
B. A higher serum IgE.
C. A higher serum IgG.
D. Increased prevalence of rheumatoid factor.
E. Increased prevalence of heterophile antibodies.

Answers overleaf

1.19 D, E

Idiotypes are antigenic determinants located in the variable part of the immunoglobulin. The so-called 'private' idiotypes include the hypervariable amino-acid residues in the antigen-binding site which have arisen by somatic mutation of genes and are unique to the individual. Other idiotypes are 'public' and coded for by germ-line genes. These therefore appear in other individuals sharing the same genes. However, unlike isotypes, all the variants of idiotypes are not present in the serum of every individual within a species. Since idiotypes can induce anti-idiotype antibody, the latter may be involved in modulation of the antibody response (Jerne's network theory).

1.20 All true

Serum IgM, IgE and IgG are higher than the normal range for Europeans. Rheumatoid factor, anti-nuclear factor, heterophile antibodies and the Wassermann reaction are more likely to be positive. Levels of immune complexes are higher. Chronic parasite infections are probably the most important factor responsible for these differences. Local normal values should always be established before interpreting immunological tests.

2. MONOCLONAL ANTIBODIES

2.1 Monoclonal antibodies are produced by the fusion of which of the
following cell types to form a hybridoma cell line?

   A. Monocyte.
   B. Lymphoma cell.
   C. Plasma cell.
   D. Activated T lymphocyte.
   E. Myeloma cell.

2.2 Fusion of the two cell types used in monoclonal antibody formation
can be induced by which of the following?

   A. Semliki Forrest virus.
   B. Polyethylene glycol.
   C. Hypoxanthine.
   D. Sendai virus.
   E. Thymidine kinase.

Answers overleaf

2.1 C, E

Myeloma cells are fused with plasma cells prepared from an immunised mouse or rat to produce a 'hybridoma' cell. This hybrid cell combines the antibody-producing properties of the plasma cell with the immortality of the myeloma tumour cell so that it will continue to grow *in vitro*. Ideally a non-synthesising, non-secreting variant of myeloma cell line is used so that any antibody secreted by the hybridoma originates from the sensitised normal plasma cell.

2.2 B, D

Polyethylene glycol or, occasionally, the Sendai virus can be used to induce fusion between myeloma and plasma cells. Plasma cells, which are terminally differentiated, die in culture, but remaining myeloma cells must be removed to select for the hybridoma cells. This can be achieved by using a myeloma cell line deficient in the enzyme responsible for incorporation of hypoxanthine into DNA. Such cells can synthesise DNA only by 'de novo' synthesis. By growing the cells in a medium containing hypoxanthine, aminopterin (which blocks 'de novo' DNA synthesis) and thymidine (HAT medium), hybridoma cells are positively selected for because the myeloma cells are unable to make DNA via the salvage pathway.

3. COMPLEMENT

3.1 Which of the following cells synthesise substantial amounts of the components of complement?

  A. Mast cells.
  B. Macrophages.
  C. Polymorphonuclear cells.
  D. Hepatocytes.
  E. Gut epithelial cells.

3.2 Which of the following is/are true concerning complement?

  A. The classical pathway can only be activated by antibody.
  B. Activation of one C1 molecule can lead to cell lysis.
  C. The alternative pathway is not dependent upon antibody for activation.
  D. It can be activated by a Gram-negative septicaemia.
  E. It is heat stable.

3.3 Which of the following immunoglobulins activates the classical complement pathway in humans?

  A. IgG1
  B. IgG4
  C. IgM
  D. IgA
  E. IgE

Answers overleaf

3.1 B, D, E

Both macrophages and the liver produce a substantial number of complement components. The only other cell type that makes substantial amounts of a complement component are the cells of the intestinal and urinary epithelium which make C1.

3.2 B, C, D

The classical pathway is essentially antibody dependent (it 'complements' antibody) but can be activated by Lipid A (from the cell wall of Gram-negative bacteria), and C-reactive protein. Activation of one C1 molecule, because it is an enzyme, activates several molecules of the next component, and so on, resulting in a cascade effect with amplification. The final result is a macroscopic event, cell lysis, as well as a number of other effects including enhancement of phagocytosis and chemotaxis. The alternative pathway is a second distinct enzyme cascade which again leads to the cleavage of C3. It is not dependent upon antibody and can therefore be activated earlier in infection, before specific antibody is present to initiate the classical pathway. Both the classical and the alternative pathways can be activated by a Gram-negative septicaemia. Complement is heat labile in contrast to antibody which is stable.

3.3 A, C

Human IgG1 and IgG3 are strong activators of the classical complement pathway. IgG2 is a weak activator and IgG4 fails to activate the classical pathway. IgM activates this pathway strongly in many species, including humans. IgA, IgG4 and IgE can in some circumstances activate the alternative pathway. IgD does not activate complement.

3.4 Concerning the classical complement pathway, which of the following is/are true?

   A. C1r is the recognition site of the C1 complex and binds to the immunoglobulin.
   B. Binding occurs between the Fab region of the immunoglobulin and C1.
   C. Activation of C1 is dependent upon magnesium ions.
   D. Activated C1 ('C1 esterase') cleaves C2 and C3.
   E. Activated C3 ('C3 convertase') cleaves C4 and C5.

3.5 Concerning C3b, which of the following is/are true?

   A. It is chemotactic to polymorphs.
   B. It is an anaphylatoxin.
   C. It enhances phagocytosis via immune adherence.
   D. It triggers the terminal membrane attack pathway of complement.
   E. It is inactivated by β1H-globulin (factor H) and C3b inactivator (factor I).

Answers overleaf

3.4 All false

The C1q component of C1 binds to the Fc region of the immunoglobulin (CH_2 domain of IgG or CH_4 domain of IgM) and, via C1r, activates C1s creating 'C1 esterase'. This is a calcium-ion-dependent process. C1 esterase cleaves C4 and C2, a magnesium-ion-dependent process, creating C$\overline{4b}$ $\overline{2a}$ which is a 'C3 convertase'. C3 convertase then 'converts' C3 to C3b and C3a fragments.

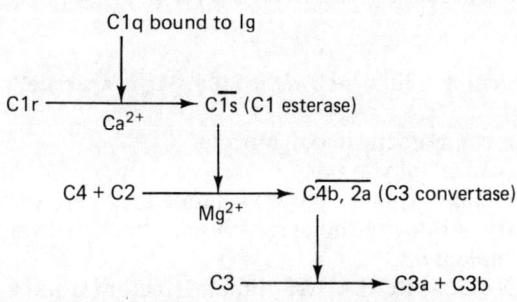

Fig. 4   The classical pathway (from C1 to C3)

3.5 C, D, E

The cleavage of C3 into C3a and C3b is the reaction at the core of the complement system. Unlike C3a and C5a, C3b is neither chemotactic nor anaphylatoxic. C3b cleaves C5 and so triggers the terminal membrane attack pathway. There are also receptors for C3b on polymorphs and macrophages. This facilitates phagocytosis of antigen–antibody–complement complexes ('immune adherence'). It can also bind to β1H-globulin (factor H) which makes it susceptible to cleavage by C3b inactivator (factor I).

3.6 Concerning the terminal stages of the complement pathway, which of the following is/are true?

A. C5 is split into C5a and C5b.
B. C5a is an anaphylatoxin and chemotactic.
C. C5b, having bound C6, 7, 8 and 9, may dissociate from the original site and bind to 'innocent' bystander cells causing cell lysis.
D. The C5–9 complex inserts itself into the membrane, causing free ion flux across it.
E. C9 is essential for cell lysis to occur.

3.7 Which of the following can activate the alternative complement pathway?

A. Bacterial endotoxins.
B. C3 nephritic factor.
C. Cryoglobulins.
D. Aggregates of IgD.
E. Cobra venom.

Answers overleaf

Complement

3.6 A, B, D

Following the formation of C3b, the terminal sequences are the same for both classical and alternative pathways and end in cell lysis. C5 is split into C5a and C5b. The former, like C3a, in anaphylatoxic, i.e. it degranulates mast cells. It is also chemotactic. C5b binds C6 and C7. This C5b, 6, 7 complex may become free and later bind to a nearby cell where, if it binds C8 and C9, it may cause lysis. Once C8 and C9 are bound the complex becomes stable. Several molecules of C9 are bound to one molecule of C5–8 forming a complex which causes free transmembrane ionic flux and cell lysis. Lysis can still occur in the absence of C9 but C9 enhances the process.

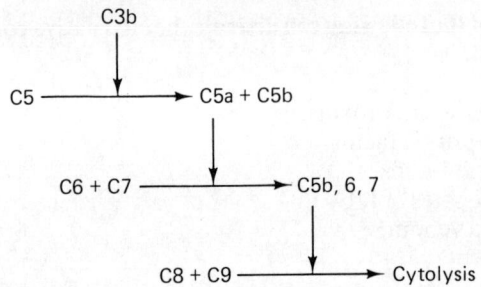

Fig. 5   The terminal complement pathway (post C3)

3.7 A, B, C, E

The alternative pathway can be activated by increasing the rate of C3b Bb formation or decreasing its rate of destruction. The polysaccharide component of bacterial endotoxins protects C3b from breakdown by β1H-globulin and C3b inactivator. The Lipid A component of bacterial endotoxins can activate the classical pathway. Cobra venom appears to be a form of C3b intrinsically resistant to breakdown by C3b inactivator. There is some evidence that cryoglobulin may act by sequestering β1H-globulin. C3 nephritic factor is an autoantibody which stabilises C3b Bb by binding to a determinant involving both parts of the complex. Aggregates of IgD do not activate complement as can, for example, aggregates of human IgA.

3.8 Which of the following is/are component(s) of the alternative complement pathway?

A. C1
B. C2
C. Factor B
D. Properdin
E. C4

3.9 A low C3 with a normal C4 level is compatible with which of the following?

A. Activation of the alternative complement pathway.
B. Membranoproliferative glomerulonephritis associated with the C3 nephritic factor.
C. Genetic deficiency of C3b inactivator.
D. Hereditary angioedema.
E. Activation of the classical complement pathway.

Answers overleaf

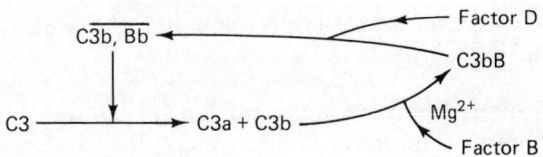

Complement

3.8 C, D

C3 can be activated by an alternative 'C3 convertase' formed from fragment b of factor B and fragment C3b. C3b binds to factor B rendering it susceptible to cleavage by factor D. Factor D splits off fragment Ba leaving C̄3̄b̄ B̄b̄, a powerful C3 convertase. This complex (C̄3̄b̄ B̄b̄) is normally unstable and rapidly broken down by C3b inactivator. However, it can be stabilised by initiators of the alternative pathway and by properdin when this is activated.

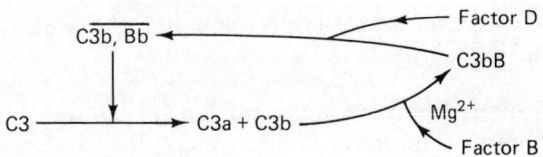

Fig. 6   The alternative pathway (note positive feedback)

3.9 A, B, C

If the early complement components, represented by C4, are normal, a low C3 suggests activation of the alternative rather than the classical pathway. In those forms of membranoproliferative glomerulonephritis with C3 nephritic factor, there is activation of the alternative pathway, and usually normal C4. However, other forms of membranoproliferative disease do occur in which both C3 and C4 are reduced. In these cases C3 nephritic factor is much less frequently detected. Genetic deficiencies of C3b inactivator and β1H microglobulin are known to exist. This leads to unrestrained activation of the alternative pathway. In contrast, deficiency of C1 esterase inhibitor (hereditary angioedema) results in a low C4 and C3. SLE is associated with a low C3 and low C4.

4. INNATE AND CELLULAR IMMUNITY

4.1 Which of the following is/are involved in innate immunity?

A. The classical complement pathway.
B. The cilia lining the respiratory tract.
C. Lysozyme.
D. IgM.
E. Neutrophils.

4.2 Which of the following is/are true concerning macrophages?

A. They can adhere to glass.
B. They can kill organisms using the myeloperoxidase–peroxide–halide system.
C. They enhance the antibody response to thymus-dependent antigens.
D. They secrete monokines.
E. They secrete lysozyme.

4.3 Which of the following cells mediate antibody-dependent cellular cytotoxicity (ADCC)?

A. B lymphocytes.
B. Basophils.
C. Eosinophils.
D. Killer (K) cells.
E. Macrophages.

Answers overleaf

4.1 B, C, E

Innate immunity refers to the non-specific mechanisms which are present before specific immunity (including IgM) can develop. They include:

1. physiochemical barriers such as the skin and mucous membranes—both mucus and cilia aid removal of bacteria,
2. bacteriocidal factors such as lysozyme which attack the bacterial cell wall; these are present in tears, nasal secretions and saliva,
3. the alternative complement pathway (the classical pathway is antibody dependent),
4. phagocytic cells such as macrophages, neutrophils and eosinophils.

4.2 A, C, D, E

Glass adherence is a useful property for separating macrophages from other cell types. Macrophages appear to ingest and kill microbes with many mechanisms similar to neutrophils but they do not use the myeloperoxidase–peroxide–halide system, which is one of the oxygen-dependent systems used by neutrophils. Ia-positive macrophages appear to enhance the antibody response to thymus-dependent antigens by processing the antigen and presenting it on the macrophage surface in a more immunogenic state. Thus it can be recognised by Ia-compatible T helper cells. Monokines are factors produced by macrophages which act on other cells, e.g. interleukin 1, colony-stimulating factor, prostaglandins. Macrophages also secrete many enzymes including lysozyme (muramidase) which is antibacterial.

4.3 C, D, E

Killer cells mediate cytotoxicity via an IgG-dependent mechanism which is not antigen specific and not MHC restricted. They are of heterogeneous cell lineage but all have IgG receptors. Eosinophils have IgE receptors and can mediate IgE-dependent cellular cytoxicity, often directed against helminths. Macrophages have IgG and IgE receptors through which they can mediate ADCC.

4.4 Which of the following human cells have Fc receptors for IgG (Fcγ)?

A. Helper T lymphocytes.
B. B lymphocytes.
C. Neutrophils.
D. Macrophages.
E. Mast cells.

4.5 Which of the following cells are phagocytic?

A. Neutrophils.
B. Eosinophils.
C. B lymphocytes.
D. T lymphocytes.
E. Kupffer cells.

4.6 Which of the following is/are true concerning Natural Killer (NK) cells?

A. They are 'spontaneously cytotoxic'.
B. Activity is major histocompatibility complex (MHC) restricted.
C. They have Fcγ receptors.
D. They are not found in athymic 'nude' mice.
E. Activity is stimulated by interferon.

Answers overleaf

4.4 B, C, D

Human helper T cells have Fcμ (IgM) receptors whereas suppressor/cytotoxic cells have Fcγ receptors. B lymphocytes, as well as expressing self-synthesised immunoglobulin, have Fcγ receptors. Their function is unknown. Macrophages and neutrophils have Fcγ receptors which mediate ADCC and facilitate phagocytosis (opsonic adherence). Macrophages, eosinophils and mast cells have Fcε (IgE) receptors. In the case of mast cells, their degranulation is initiated by stimulation of cell-bound IgE.

4.5 A, B, E

Phagocytosis is the process of engulfment of material into a cell. The material is enclosed in a protoplasmic invagination, 'the phagosome', and then digested by lysosomal enzymes. Neutrophils and eosinophils ('microphages') are good phagocytes as are cells of the macrophage cell line—Kupffer cells (liver), monocytes (blood), histiocytes (tissues), microglial cells (central nervous system) and osteoclasts (bone). Neutrophils, eosinophils and macrophages have Fc and C3b receptors which can enhance phagocytosis of antibody-coated (opsonic adherence) or complement-coated (immune adherence) organisms.

4.6 A, C, E

'Natural Killer' cells are thus named because they are spontaneously cytotoxic against many tumour and virally infected cells *in vitro*. They cause cell death in the absence of both antibody- and antigen-specific stimulation. However, they do have Fcγ receptors and probably overlap with 'K' (Killer) cells which mediate ADCC. Their exact cell lineage is uncertain. They have some T-cell markers but are not dependent on the presence of a thymus and are present in 'nude' athymic mice. Their activity is not MHC restricted. Activity is stimulated by interferon and, *in vivo*, NK cells probably play an important role in the killing of tumour cells. Their cytolytic activity shows some selectivity in that not all target cells are equally susceptible to NK cells from different donors.

4.7 Which of the following is/are true concerning human suppressor T lymphocytes?

   A. They are present in the circulation in greater numbers than helper T cells.
   B. They bear OKT4 antigen.
   C. They are distinguished from cytotoxic T cells by the presence of Leu 2a antigen.
   D. They can be activated by concanavalin A.
   E. They suppress T helper cells.

4.8 Which of the following is/are true concerning typical T lymphocytes located in the cortex of the murine thymus?

   A. They express the TL antigen.
   B. They have high levels of Thy-1(θ) antigen.
   C. They have high levels of H-2 antigens.
   D. They are cortisone resistant.
   E. They are small, dense and short lived.

4.9 In which of the following tissues are over 60% of the lymphocytes B cells?

   A. The peripheral blood.
   B. The thoracic duct.
   C. The spleen.
   D. The lymph nodes.
   E. The thymus.

4.10 Which of the following is/are true concerning murine cytotoxic T lymphocytes?

   A. They can lyse cells bearing allogenic H-2K and D antigens.
   B. They can lyse virally infected syngeneic cells.
   C. They are antigen specific.
   D. They require specific antibody to mediate cell lysis.
   E. They can revert to small memory T cells.

Answers overleaf

4.7 D, E

Suppressor T cells are present in lower numbers than T helper cells. Both cytotoxic and suppressor T cells bear OKT5, 8 and Leu 2a antigens. Helper T cells are OKT4 and Leu 3a positive. Suppressor T cells suppress T helper cells and B lymphocyte antibody responses. Tolerance induced by low antigen concentrations may be mediated by T-cell suppression of T helper cells. Concanavalin A non-specifically activates suppressor cells at certain concentrations.

4.8 A, B, E

Ninety per cent of small lymphocytes in the thymus are small, dense, short-lived lymphocytes expressing TL antigen, high levels of Thy-1 antigen and low levels of H-2 antigens. They are cortisone sensitive and located predominantly in the cortex. More mature T lymphocytes are located in the medulla of the thymus and differ in being slightly larger and less dense, cortisone resistant and TL-antigen negative. They bear higher levels of histocompatibility antigens and lower levels of Thy-1 antigen.

4.9 C

In man 70–80% of peripheral blood lymphocytes are T cells and 15–20% B cells; 80% of lymphocytes in the lymph nodes and 85% in the thoracic duct are T cells. B lymphocytes are in the majority in the spleen, where about 35% of lymphocytes are T cells.

4.10 A, B, C, E

Cytotoxic T lymphocytes can specifically lyse allogenic cells carrying foreign H-2K and D antigens or syngeneic H-2 identical cells bearing viral surface antigens. Cytolysis is antigen specific and involves direct contact between T lymphocyte and target cell. It is not antibody dependent. Cytotoxic T lymphocytes can revert to memory cells.

4.11 Mice thymectomised within 48 hours of birth demonstrate which of the following?

  A. Low serum IgG levels.
  B. A decrease in circulating lymphocytes.
  C. A decreased ability to reject skin grafts.
  D. Normal humoral response to all antigens.
  E. Severe wasting.

4.12 Which of the following areas is/are thymus dependent?

  A. The cortical region of the lymph node.
  B. The medullary region of the lymph node.
  C. The paracortical zone of the lymph node.
  D. The lymphocytic periarteriolar sheaths in the spleen.
  E. The lymphoid nodules in the spleen.

4.13 A mouse is challenged for the first time with intravenous pneumococcal polysaccharide. Four days later a lymph node taken at autopsy is likely to show which of the following changes?

  A. Large numbers of plasma cells in the germinal centres of the lymphoid follicles.
  B. Lymphocyte proliferation and plasma cells in the medullary region.
  C. Intense lymphocyte proliferation in the paracortical region.
  D. Location of antigen primarily in the macrophages of the medullary zone.
  E. Location of antigen primarily in the dendritic reticular cells of the germinal centres.

Answers overleaf

4.11 B, C, E

If a mouse is thymectomised within 48 hours of birth, there is a marked diminution in circulating lymphocytes over the next 2–3 months. There is also severe impairment of graft rejection and delayed hypersensitivity reactions. This reflects the cessation of development of T-cell-mediated immunity. Humoral immunity is not directly affected, as indicated by the normal or increased immunoglobulin levels. However, the antibody response to some antigens (e.g. sheep erythrocytes) is impaired because it is dependent upon T lymphocyte co-operation with B cells ('thymus-dependent antigens'). Severe wasting occurs, possibly due to multiple infections. If thymectomy is postponed to the third postnatal day, these disastrous effects do not occur, presumably because the secondary lymphoid organs soon become relatively self-sufficient.

4.12 C, D

The peripheral cortical region, with the lymphoid follicles, and the central medullary zone of the lymph node are thymus-independent areas containing B lymphocytes. T lymphocytes are located mainly in the paracortical region, an ill-defined intermediate area between the cortex and medulla. The lymphocytes in this area disappear after thymectomy and it is therefore 'thymus dependent'. In the spleen, the lymphocytic periarteriolar sheath is thymus dependent, whereas the lymphoid nodules contain B lymphocytes.

4.13 B, D

Most antigens induce changes in both thymus-dependent and thymus-independent areas but pneumococcal polysaccharide is a thymus-independent antigen and therefore the paracortical area is uninvolved. Lymphocyte proliferation and the development of plasma cells occur in the medullary zone and antigen is encountered in the macrophages of this area. In secondary responses, involvement of the germinal centres is much more marked and develops rapidly, with intense lymphocyte proliferation, plasma cell formation and location of much of the antigen in the dendritic reticular cells of this area. Thus **E** refers to a secondary response.

4.14 The surface of human T lymphocytes is characterised by the presence of which of the following?

A. Thy-I(θ) antigen.
B. Receptors for sheep erythrocytes.
C. Surface immunoglobulin on some cells.
D. C3 receptors.
E. Receptors for mouse erythrocytes.

4.15 Concerning murine T lymphocyte surface phenotype, which of the following is/are true?

A. They bear receptors for sheep erythrocytes.
B. The Ly b series of antigens is present.
C. Qa-I-positive cells are involved in the generation of suppressor cells.
D. Ia-positive cells are not detectable.
E. Thy-I (θ) antigen is acquired before reaching the thymus.

4.16 The surface phenotype of human B lymphocytes is characterised by the presence of which of the following?

A. Epstein Barr virus (EBV) receptors.
B. Measles receptors.
C. OKT antigens.
D. C3 receptors.
E. Receptors for mouse erythrocytes.

4.17 Interleukin 2 (T-cell growth factor) is produced by which of the following?

A. Macrophages.
B. B lymphocytes.
C. Lyt 1+ T lymphocytes.
D. Lymphocytes stimulated by pokeweed mitogen.
E. Lymphocytes stimulated by alloantigens.

Answers overleaf

4.14 B, C

Only murine T cells have Thy-I antigen. Human T lymphocytes can be distinguished from B cells by their ability to form E rosettes with sheep erythrocytes. Surface immunoglobulin is detectable on some T cells due to adsorbtion via Fc receptors. Human T lymphocytes do not have receptors for C3 or mouse erythrocytes.

4.15 C

Unlike human T cells, murine T lymphocytes do not form rosettes with sheep erythrocytes. They bear the Ly t series of antigens, while B cells carry the Ly b antigens. Qa-1-positive helper cells are involved in the generation of T suppressor cells, whereas Qa-I-negative helper cells co-operate with B cells. Ia antigens are detectable on activated T lymphocytes. The Thy-I antigen is acquired by murine T cells in the thymus.

4.16 A, D, E

Human B cells have receptors for EBV, mouse erythrocytes and C3 receptors. Human T lymphocytes have receptors for measles virus and bear the OKT series of antigens.

4.17 C, E

Interleukin 2 (IL2) is produced by T lymphocytes stimulated by T cell lectins such as phytohaemagglutinins or T-dependent antigens (e.g. alloantigens). Pokeweed mitogen stimulates B cells. IL2 is produced predominantly by the Lyt 1+ helper subset in mice. In man, both T helper cells and T suppressor/cytotoxic cells can produce IL2 in response to mitogens, but after allogeneic stimulation IL2 production is predominantly from the helper subset.

4.18 Concerning interleukin 2, which of the following is/are true?

A. It is antigen specific.
B. It has no detectable effect on unprimed T cells.
C. It is major histocompatibility complex (MHC) restricted.
D. DNA synthesis is required for its production.
E. It can be used *in vitro* to derive clones of T cells from a single progenitor cell in the absence of macrophages.

4.19 Concerning interleukin 1, which of the following is/are true?

A. It is produced by B lymphocytes.
B. It stimulates proliferation of unprimed T lymphocytes.
C. Activity is antigen specific.
D. It induces the synthesis and secretion of lymphokines by T cells.
E. It is a protein of 30 000 d.

4.20 Concerning the bursa of Fabricius, which of the following is/are true?

A. It is an example of a secondary lymphoid organ.
B. It contains many proliferating lymphocytes during fetal development.
C. It contains lymphocytes whose proliferation is mainly antigen dependent.
D. It is found only in birds, located near the cloaca.
E. It consists of many epithelial folds, similar in structure to the lobules of the thymus.

Answers overleaf

4.18 B

Interleukin 2 (IL2) activity is not antigen specific and not MHC restricted. T cells appear to acquire receptors for IL2 after activation by antigen or mitogen and IL2 does not appear to affect unprimed lymphocytes. IL2 has been used to derive clones of T lymphocytes from single progenitor cells *in vitro* but magrophages ('feeder cells') must also be present for this to succeed. IL2 can be produced by non-dividing cells provided that protein synthesis is intact.

4.19 D

Interleukin 1 (IL1) is produced by macrophages. Like IL2, it has no effect on unprimed T lymphocytes and its activity is not antigen specific. It stimulates activated T cells to proliferate and to produce lymphokines and IL2. Murine IL2 has a molecular weight of about 30 000 d whereas IL1 has a molecular weight of about 15 000 d.

4.20 B, D, E

The bursa of Fabricius, like the thymus, is a primary lymphoid organ, containing rapidly dividing lymphocytes during fetal development. This proliferation is antigen independent. In contrast, lymphopoiesis in secondary lymphoid organs is antigen dependent and only becomes evident after birth when the neonate comes into contact with foreign antigens. The bursa of Fabricius is structurally similar to the thymus and is found in birds near the cloaca. Its epithelial component 'educates' the antibody-producing B lymphocytes. Its mammalian equivalent is unknown.

Innate and Cellular Immunity

4.21 Mast cells granules contain which of the following?

  A. Myeloperoxidase.
  B. Heparin.
  C. Histamine.
  D. Eosinophil chemotactic factor.
  E. Slow-reacting substances of anaphylaxis (SRS-A).

4.22 A secondary antibody response to the hapten dinitrophenyl (DNP) is likely if a mouse primed with DNP-BSA (bovine serum albumin carrier) is challenged with which of the following?

  A. DNP-BSA.
  B. DNP-OVA (ovalbumin carrier).
  C. 4-hydroxy-3-iodo-5-nitrophenacetyl (NIP)-BSA.
  D. BSA and DNP-OVA.
  E. Further primed with OVA and then challenged with DNP-OVA.

Answers overleaf

4.21 B, C, D, E

The metachromatic granules of mast cells contain heparin, histamine, eosinophil chemotactic factor, SRS-A, prostaglandins, platelet-activating factor (PAF), sulphated mucopolysaccharides and a large number of enzymes but not myeloperoxidase. Myeloperoxidase is present in neutrophil granules.

4.22 A, E

A secondary antibody response to the hapten only occurs when lymphocytes are primed to both hapten and carrier (hence **B** and **C** fail). The T cells then recognise the carrier and help the B cells in producing antibody to the hapten. T cell co-operation permits the switch from IgM to IgG synthesis. The carrier (BSA) and the hapten (DNP) must be on the same antigen molecule (**A**) to evoke a secondary response, hence challenge with BSA and DNP-OVA fails. However, if the DNP-BSA-primed mouse is further primed with OVA before challenge with DNP-OVA, a secondary response occurs.

5. INTERFERON

5.1 Which of the following is/are true concerning interferon?

A. It is always non-antigenic in the homologous host.
B. It can be produced by lymphocytes as part of the cell-mediated response.
C. It is non-dialysable.
D. It is a glycoprotein.
E. It has a molecular weight of 200 000 d.

5.2 Which of the following is/are true concerning interferon α?

A. There are 14 subtypes.
B. It can be derived from the buffy coat of fresh blood following stimulation by Sendai virus.
C. Each subtype is a product of one gene.
D. There is up to 30% difference in amino acid sequences between subtypes.
E. It is acid stable.

5.3. Which of the following is/are true concerning interferon β?

A. It is known as fibroblast interferon.
B. There are 5 subtypes.
C. It is acid labile.
D. It is induced by poly I poly C.
E. It is induced by carboxymethylcellulose.

Answers overleaf

5.1 B, C, D

Interferon comprises a small molecular-weight (about 20 000–35 000 d) non-dialysable group of glycoproteins. Additional higher molecular weight species are now thought to be contaminants. It is usually non-antigenic in the homologous host but neutralising antibodies have been induced in the homologous host when interferon has been used in treatment. It possesses both antiviral and antitumour properties.

5.2 All true

Interferon α exists in 14 subtypes and each is the product of one gene. It can be induced by viruses such as Sendai and Newcastle disease viruses. It is thought that the different subtypes started to evolve from each other about 80 million years ago. Interferon α is also called leucocyte interferon.

5.3 A, D, E

There is one type of interferon β and it is produced by fibroblasts in response to poly I poly C or carboxymethylcellulose. It is acid stable, like interferon α. It is thought to have evolved from interferon α 200 million years ago. It can be produced by stimulation of T cell lines by virus.

Interferon

5.4 Which of the following is/are true concerning interferon γ?

   A. It is produced in response to viruses.
   B. It is produced in response to antigenic stimulation.
   C. It is acid labile.
   D. It shows 30% DNA homology with interferon α.
   E. It shows 30% DNA homology with interferon β.

5.5 Which of the following is/are true concerning interferon?

   A. It can activate Natural Killer cells.
   B. It enhances T-cell cytotoxicity.
   C. It activates macrophages.
   D. It can induce 2-5 A synthetase.
   E. It can induce a protein kinase.

5.6 The side-effects of interferon include which of the following?

   A. Pyrexia.
   B. Granulocytopenia.
   C. Peripheral sensory neuropathy.
   D. Extreme confusion.
   E. Hypotension.

5.7 Which of the following tumours has/have shown some response to interferon?

   A. Lymphocytic lymphomas.
   B. Histiocytic lymphomas.
   C. IgA-producing malignant myelomas.
   D. IgG-producing malignant myelomas.
   E. Bronchial carcinomas.

Answers overleaf

5.4 B, C

Interferon γ differs from α and β by being acid labile and it is not produced in response to viruses. It is produced by T lymphocytes in mixed cell culture with macrophages. It is induced by mitogens such as phytohaemagglutinin. It shows only minor DNA homology with interferon α, and none with interferon β.

5.5 All true

Interferon is a lymphokine which can activate Natural Killer cells, T cell cytoxicity, B-cell antibody production and macrophages. It can induce a protein kinase enzyme in response to double-stranded RNA. This phosphorylates a subunit in interferon α. The phosphorylated form leads to inhibition of protein synthesis by blocking the initiating complex. Interferon also induces a 2–5 A synthetase. This leads to production of 2–5 A, a group of oligonucleotides which activate an endonuclease which can degrade foreign mRNA (e.g. viral).

5.6 All true

Interferon produces pyrexia which is reversed by aspirin and usually abates with continued treatment. It produces anorexia, fatigue, weight loss, granulocytopenia (usually reversible), raised serum aminotransferases, arthralgia, myalgia, hypotension, headaches, hair shedding, peripheral sensory neuropathy and confusion. The confusion is induced by the higher doses and correlates with EEC changes. It was originally thought these side-effects were due to impurities included during interferon production. Now that pure interferon is available by cloning, it has been shown that the pure compound in pharmacological doses is highly toxic.

5.7 A, C

Lymphocytic lymphomas respond but histiocytic lymphomas do not. IgA and Bence–Jones-producing malignant myelomas respond to interferon at a comparable rate to melphalon. The IgG-producing type do not seem to respond. Laryngeal papillomas also show some response.

6. THE MAJOR HISTOCOMPATIBILITY COMPLEX

6.1 Which of the following is/are true concerning the major histocompatibility complex (MHC) in mammals?

    A. It is found in all mammals.
    B. In the mouse it is located on chromosome 18.
    C. Its primary function is the rejection of foreign transplants.
    D. Transplant survival is determined by immune response (Ir) genes.
    E. Transplant rejection is determined by major histocompatibility antigens.

6.2 Which of the following is/are true concerning the MHC in man?

    A. It is located on the long arm of chromosome 6.
    B. It constitutes 4% of the total genome.
    C. It is called the H-2 system.
    D. Autografts carry identical MHC antigens.
    E. It is the basis of Jerne's network theory.

6.3 The H-2 locus contains genes coding for which of the following?

    A. H-2A antigens.
    B. H-2I antigens.
    C. H-2B antigens.
    D. The C4 component of complement.
    E. All the transplantation antigens.

Answers overleaf

6.1 A, E

The major histocompatibility complex (MHC) is found in all mammals and is relatively homologous between species. It is on chromosome 17 in the mouse. Its primary function is in immune regulation but it was originally discovered through transplantation experiments. Transplant survival is primarily influenced by the presence of MHC antigens and not immune response genes.

6.2 D

The MHC in man is situated on the short arm of chromosome 6 and constitutes 0.4% of the total genome. It is called the HLA system in man and H-2 in mouse. Autografts are between self and self. They are therefore by definition MHC identical. Jerne's network theory is based on idiotype–anti-idiotype interactions and not MHC restriction.

6.3 B, D

The H-2 locus, found in the mouse, contains K, I, C4, D, L, Qa, and TL regions. There exist other transplant antigens outside the major histocompatibility complex locus.

6.4 Which of the following is/are true concerning the H-2 locus?

A. K and D code for the classical transplantation antigens.
B. K and D antigens are defined using the mixed lymphocyte reaction.
C. The I region has been subdivided into regions A, J, E, and C.
D. I-B was previously thought to be a subset of I but is no longer thought to exist.
E. L codes for a minor series of transplantation antigens.

6.5 The HLA locus contains genes coding for which of the following?

A. The C4 component of complement.
B. The C2 component of complement.
C. Factor B.
D. HLA-B antigens.
E. HLA-C antigens, the locus being between the A and B regions.

6.6 Concerning allotypes, which of the following is/are true?

A. They are idiotypes which behave as xenotypes in other individuals of the same species.
B. They fail to elicit specific antibodies in some other members of the species of origin.
C. They differ from each other antigenically.
D. They are those isotypes which behave as autotypes in other individuals of the same species.
E. They are antigens which stimulate a Type I allergic reaction.

6.7 Which of the following is/are true concerning Class I proteins in man?

A. They are only found on lymphocytes.
B. They are a subset of Class II.
C. They are controlled by the K, D and L regions.
D. They are controlled by the Ia region.
E. They are important in complement activation.

Answers overleaf

6.4 A, C, D, E

H-2 K and D code for the classical transplantation antigens which are serologically defined using alloantisera. The mixed lymphocyte reaction defines 'lymphocyte-activating determinants', coded for by the I region. The I region is at present subdivided into A, J, E, and C. I-B is no longer thought to exist. There has recently been some doubt as to the existence of I-J. L codes for a minor series of transplantation antigens, structurally similar to K and D.

6.5 All true

The HLA system is found in man and consists of a Dr region followed by regions coding for C4, C2, factor B and the Chido and Rogers blood groups. Finally there is HLA-B, C and then A. This is reading away from the centromere.

6.6 A, B, C

Alleles are inherited variants at a genetic locus. Allotypes are the products of alleles and are inherited antigenic variants of a particular molecule. Allotypes of a single protein thus differ from each other antigenically. They also fail to elicit antibodies in members of the same species with identical allotype. In Jerne's terminology, allotypes are those idiotypes (i.e. antigenic specificities) which behave as xenotypes (i.e. as if they are from another species) in other individuals of the same species. Allotypes do not stimulate Type I allergic reactions. Isotypes contrast to alloytpes in that they are the same for all normal individuals of the same animal species.

6.7 All false

Class I molecules are found on essentially all cells. They are independent of Class II and are controlled, in man, by the HLA-A, B and C loci. They have nothing to do with complement activation.

6.8 **Which of the following is/are true concerning Class I proteins in the mouse?**

A. They are found on leucocytes.
B. They are a subset of Class III.
C. They are controlled by the K, D and L regions.
D. They are controlled by the Ia region.
E. They are recognised by cytotoxic T cells.

6.9 **In man, Class II molecules differ from Class I in which of the following ways?**

A. They are important in interactions between macrophages and T cells.
B. They are important in interactions between T and B lymphocytes.
C. They restrict suppressor T cell activity.
D. They activate complement.
E. They are linked to HLA-Dr.

6.10 **Class III molecules are concerned with which of the following?**

A. C4 and C3 in mice.
B. C4, C2 and factor B in man.
C. Transplant rejection.
D. B cell idiotypes.
E. T cells.

6.11 **Alloantisera, in humans, can be derived from which of the following?**

A. People who have had multiple blood transfusions.
B. Multiparous women.
C. Immunised human volunteers.
D. Immunised thymectomised mice.
E. People who have rejected a kidney transplant.

Answers overleaf

6.8 A, C, E

Class I proteins are independent of Class III and are controlled by the K, D and L loci in the mouse. They are found on essentially all cells, including leucocytes. They are recognised by cytotoxic T cells.

6.9 A, B, C, E

Class II molecules are linked to HLA-Dr (man) and H-2 I and E (mouse). They are responsible for the mixed lymphocyte reaction. Interactions between macrophages and T helper cells and between the latter and B lymphocytes are restricted or 'guided' by a need for compatibility between Class II antigens. T suppressor cells are restricted by Class II (J) antigens. Cytotoxic T cells are restricted by Class I, not Class II, antigens. Activation of complement is a Class III function.

6.10 A, B

Class III molecules have nothing to do with B cell idiotypes. They code for certain components of complement (C4 and C3 in mice, C4, C2 and factor B in man) and the Chido and Rogers blood groups. They have no relevance to cellular cytotoxicity.

6.11 A, B, C, E

Antisera produced by injecting animals with antigens obtained from a different species are termed xenoantisera (from Greek *xenos* = foreign). On the other hand, antigens detected by immunisation of different individuals within the same species are called alloantigens and the antisera obtained are called alloantisera (from the Greek *allos* = the other). In the immunised mouse, any antibody produced would be an example of a xenoantiserum as regards man.

6.12 Concerning the term linkage disequilibrium, which of the following is/are true?

A. It refers to the unequal numbers of B and T cells in the circulation.
B. It describes a situation in which the frequency of the combination of two alleles is higher or lower than expected.
C. It describes a situation in which the frequency of the combination of two alleles is equal to that predicted.
D. It is a phenomenon restricted to the MHC genes.
E. It occurs with HLA–A1 and B8 in humans.

6.13 Concerning the structure of HLA-A and B antigens, which of the following is/are true?

A. They comprise three polypeptides.
B. They contain a β_2-microglobulin.
C. They contain a heavy chain with a single asparagine-linked oligosaccharide unit.
D. They contain a heavy chain which traverses the lipid cellular bilayer once.
E. There is a hydrophilic domain at the carboxy terminus.

6.14 Concerning the β_2-microglobulin in man, which of the following is/are true?

A. It carries the allotypic determinants.
B. It is non-glycosylated.
C. It is coded for by a gene on chromosome 15.
D. It shows striking homology between its amino acid sequence and the third constant region domain of the heavy chain of IgG.
E. It has a molecular weight of 44 000 d.

6.15 Concerning HLA-Dr antigens, which of the following is/are true?

A. They are composed of three polypeptides.
B. The molecular weights of these are 34 000, 28 000 and 10 000 d.
C. The polypeptides are non-glycosylated.
D. The polypeptides are loosely associated.
E. The α chain is unphosphorylated. *Answers overleaf*

49

6.12 B, E

Linkage disequilibrium describes a situation in which the frequency of the combination of two alleles is higher or lower than expected. An allele is an inherited variant at a particular locus. One example is the association of HLA-A1 and B8. The associations are thought either to reflect some evolutionary advantage or to be due to the fact that insufficient generations have passed for the two characters to become separated. The phenomenon is not restricted to the MHC.

6.13 B, C, D, E

HLA-A and B antigens comprise two polypeptide chains. The heavy chain represents the HLA-A and B gene product. It possesses a single asparagine-linked oligosaccharide unit and crosses the lipid bilayer once. There is a hydrophilic domain at the carboxy terminus with a high serine content. The other chain is the β_2-microglobulin.

6.14 B, C, D

β_2-microglobulin has a molecular weight of 11 600 d, whereas that of the heavy chain is 44 000 d. The heavy chain carries the allotypic determinants. β_2-microglobulin is non-glycosylated, coded by chromosome 15 and shows striking homology with the third constant region domain of the heavy chain of IgG.

6.15 All false

HLA-Dr antigens (Class II) comprise two polypeptide chains of molecular weights about 34 000 d (α chain) and 28 000 d (β chain). They are both glycosylated and tightly associated. The α chain is phosphorylated at its carboxy end.

6.16 **Concerning the cleavage of the HLA-B7 antigen by papain, which of the following is/are true?**

A. The papain-cleaved fragment has two disulphide-bonded loops.
B. The site of cleavage is intracellular.
C. The β_2-microglobulin portion is preferentially removed from the α chain.
D. The site of cleavage varies from cell to cell.
E. The water-soluble fragment retains alloantigenicity.

6.17 **Concerning the structure of the HLA-A or B molecule, which of the following is/are true?**

A. It is comprised of four domains on the external surface of the lipid bilayer.
B. The heavy chain forms the α, β and γ domains.
C. The C-terminal is intracellular.
D. A hydrophilic area crosses the plasma membrane.
E. The N-terminal is hydrophilic.

6.18 **Concerning the HLA-Dr, which of the following is/are true?**

A. It is defined by the mixed lymphocyte reaction (MLR).
B. It is defined by a serological reaction using antisera that have been absorbed with platelets to remove antibodies to HLA-A, B and C.
C. It is synonymous with HLA-D.
D. It is synonymous with HLA-C.
E. It is a determinant on B lymphocytes and macrophages analogous to the Ia determinant in mice.

Answers overleaf

6.16 A, E

Papain cleaves the Class I HLA-B7 molecule extracellularly, close to the plasma membrane. This occurs at a constant position, producing a water-soluble fragment of molecular weight 34 000 d. This fragment retains alloantigenicity. It contains two disulphide-bonded loops.

6.17 A, C, E

The molecule consists of four domains on the external surface of the plasma membrane. The heavy chain forms the $\alpha 1$, $\alpha 2$ and $\alpha 3$ domains. The β_2-microglobulin comprises the final domain. Both the C-terminal (intracellular) and N-terminal (extracellular) are hydrophilic. The small portion of the molecule which crosses the plasma membrane is hydrophobic.

6.18 B, E

HLA-Dr is defined serologically by antisera absorbed with platelets to remove antibodies to Class I antigens. It is present on B lymphocytes and macrophages and analogous to the Ia determinant in mice. HLA-D is defined by the mixed lymphocyte reaction. There is a good but not complete correlation between HLA-Dr and HLA-D.

6.19 A mouse is infected with lymphochoriomeningitis virus and the lymphocytes are subsequently removed. They are incubated *in vitro* with peritoneal cells radioactively labelled with chromium-51 (^{51}Cr). Free ^{51}Cr is detected in the supernatant after 8 hours. Which of the following is/are true?

A. The presence of free ^{51}Cr indicates cell lysis.

B. The ^{51}Cr-labelled peritoneal cells must be from a mouse previously infected with lymphocytic choriomeningitis virus.

C. The ^{51}Cr-labelled peritoneal cells must have the same Class I alleles as the lymphocytes.

D. The ^{51}Cr-labelled peritoneal cells must be from exactly the same mouse.

E. The ^{51}Cr-labelled peritoneal cells must have the same Ia antigen.

6.20 Which of the following is/are true?

A. Tandem duplication refers to the recycling of genetic material within an individual.

B. There are probably 20–50 genes in the major histocompatibility complex involved in peptide production.

C. There is a 1 in 4 chance of two siblings having identical HLA specificities.

D. The major histocompatibility system in the rat is referred to as RTI.

E. The major histocompatibility system in the rhesus monkey is referred to as DLA.

Answers overleaf

6.19 A, B, C

The presence of free ^{51}Cr indicates lysis of the peritoneal cells, which must be from a mouse infected by the same virus and sharing the same Class I alleles. In other words, the target cells and the cytotoxic T lymphocytes must share the same K or D allele. They do not need to have identical Ia (Class II) antigens and may come from a different mouse. The effector cell is a Ly-2+ 3+ T lymphocyte.

6.20 B, C, D

Tandem duplication refers to the idea that one primordial gene, by duplication and modification, is responsible for the HLA system. There are about 20–50 genes in the MHC involved in peptide production. Each HLA haplotype is inherited *en bloc* so that there is a 1 in 4 chance of two siblings having identical HLA specificities. The MHC in the rat is referred to as RTI, in the dog it is DLA and in the rhesus monkey it is referred to as RhLA.

7. HYPERSENSITIVITY AND DRUG ALLERGY

7.1 Concerning Type 1 reactions, which of the following is/are true?

A. Major histocompatibility complex restriction is important.
B. Low levels of neonatal gut IgA may predispose to sensitisation.
C. Platelet-activating factor may play a role.
D. IgA is the most important immunoglobulin in the reaction.
E. Mediators include tissue basophils and blood mast cells.

7.2 Concerning the Prausnitz–Kustner reaction, which of the following is/are true?

A. It is a test for reagins in atopic patients.
B. It is a passive transfer test.
C. It is a precipitation reaction.
D. It is sensitive to serum dilutions of 1:16 000.
E. It does not carry a risk of transfer of hepatitis B virus.

7.3 Concerning anaphylactoid reactions, which of the following is/are true?

A. The reaction may occur following primary exposure.
B. Sensitisation is unimportant.
C. Mediators include histamine.
D. Mediators exclude IgE.
E. Examples include strawberry allergy.

Answers overleaf

7.1 B, C

Type 1 reactions are mediated via IgE by tissue mast cells and blood basophils. These cells degranulate in response to a combination of antigen with the cell-bound IgE, releasing secondary mediators, e.g. platelet-activating factor. Low gut IgA allows larger quantities of ingested antigens to reach the circulation and induce IgE. This may predispose to Type 1 hypersensitivity reactions.

7.2 A, B, D

This reaction is a passive transfer test for reaginic antibody (IgE) in atopic individuals. Serum from an allergic patient is injected intradermally into a non-allergic recipient. If positive, the patch of skin injected becomes sensitised to the IgE–mast-cell-mediated response to the original antigen. As in any procedures involving transfer of serum between individuals, hepatitis B can be transferred.

7.3 All true

Anaphylactoid reactions differ from anaphylactic reactions in that they are independent of IgE and involve release of the same mediators by direct action on the mast cells. Prior sensitisation is therefore unimportant and the reaction may follow primary exposure. Strawberries precipitate anaphylactoid reactions in some individuals.

7.4 Concerning anaphylaxis due to drugs, which of the following is/are true?

A. It can be caused by oral administration.
B. It is most severe during the first contact between drug and patient.
C. It can be mimicked by a bee sting.
D. It should be proven clinically by rechallenging the patient.
E. It is always a Type I reaction.

7.5 Concerning Type II reactions, which of the following is/are true?

A. The antigen is bound to the cell surface.
B. Killer cells are sometimes activated.
C. Immune complexes are deposited in the kidney.
D. Complement is always activated.
E. The consequences depend on the anatomical site of the target.

7.6 Which of the following is/are NOT Type II reaction(s)?

A. Goodpasture's syndrome.
B. Sedormid-induced haemolytic anaemia.
C. Asthma.
D. Myasthenia gravis.
E. Incompatible blood transfusions.

7.7 Which of the following is/are important in the pathogenesis of Type III reactions?

A. Complement activation.
B. Platelet aggregation.
C. Local ischaemia.
D. Lysis of innocent bystander cells.
E. Polymorphonuclear chemotaxis.

Answers overleaf

7.4 A, C, E

Anaphylaxis, by definition, is a Type I reaction. It requires prior sensitisation and hence occurs on second and subsequent contacts. Anaphylactic reactions can be precipitated by second exposure to certain drugs (oral or parenteral) in sensitive individuals. In others, the same reaction can be caused by a bee sting.

7.5 A, B, E

In Type II reactions the antigen involved is bound to the cell surface. The consequences therefore depend on the site of the target antigen. Killer cells (K cells) are sometimes activated and complement may or may not be activated. Immune complex deposition is a feature of Type III reactions.

7.6 C

In Type II reactions the antigen is bound to the cell surface. In Goodpasture's syndrome this is the glomerular basement membrane; in sedormid-induced haemolytic anaemia and incompatible blood transfusions, it is the red blood cell. In the case of sedormid, the sedormid acts as a hapten and sensitises the host to its own erythrocytes. In myasthenia gravis the target is the acetylcholine receptor in the neuromuscular junction. In all the above, antibody is produced to a specific cellular-bound antigen or group of antigens. In asthma this is not so and the reaction is more of a Type I reaction in nature.

7.7 All true

The basis of the Type III reaction is formation of the antigen–antibody immune complex. These complexes can produce a variety of biological effects. They can activate complement leading to the production of chemotactic, anaphylactic and cell lytic components. They can cause platelet aggregation leading to microthrombi and local ischaemia. Chemotactically attracted neutrophils may cause further local tissue damage by releasing proteases, kinins and vasoactive amines.

7.8 Concerning circulating immune complexes, which of the following is/are true?

    A. The larger the complex, the longer the survival time in circulation.
    B. Extravascular complexes are cleared more easily than intravascular.
    C. They are precipitated by low concentrations of polyethylene glycol.
    D. During formation there is a change in immunoglobulin surface charge.
    E. They localise in capillary networks.

7.9 Which of the following is/are example(s) of Type III reaction(s) in which antigen is in excess?

    A. Serum sickness.
    B. Farmer's lung.
    C. Glomerulonephritis due to chronic antigen–antibody complex deposition.
    D. The Arthus reaction.
    E. Jarisch–Herxheimer reaction.

7.10 Which of the following is/are true concerning the Arthus reaction?

    A. Sensitivity can be passively transferred.
    B. It can be depressed by corticosteroid administration.
    C. Macroscopic changes appear in the skin after 2–4 days.
    D. Lysosomal enzymes from neutrophils cause most tissue damage.
    E. IgD is an important reaction modulator.

Answers overleaf

7.8 C, D, E

Larger complexes are removed more quickly than smaller ones by the reticuloendothelial system. Intravascular complexes are easier to clear than extravascular as it is in this compartment that most of the phagocytic cells exist. During complex formation there is a change in surface charge. Precipitation is best achieved by low concentrations of polyethylene glycol. Complexes tend to localise in capillary networks.

7.9 A, C, E

Type III reactions can be subdivided into those in which antibody is in excess (the Arthus reaction) and those where antigen is in excess. Antigen excess can be acute (serum sickness) or chronic (antigen–antibody complex disease). The Jarisch–Herxheimer reaction is an example of acute antigen excess. When syphilis is treated by penicillin there is initially a large release of antigen from dead spirochaetes. A low-grade pyrexia is often associated with myalgia, headache and malaise. The skin leasons of secondary syphilis are often exacerbated. The exact pathogenesis is unclear but there is some evidence for complement activation. Farmer's lung is an example of an Arthus reaction.

7.10 A, B, D

The Arthus reaction occurs in antibody excess and is thus restricted to where antigen first encounters antibody. An example is Farmer's lung in which inhaled antigen encounters an antibody excess in the lung alveoli. This leads to complement activation and neutrophil chemotaxis. Damage is due largely to the release of lysosomal enzymes from neutrophils and occurs in 2–4 hours. Sensitivity can be passively transferred, and is steroid responsive. IgD has no role to play.

7.11 Which of the following is/are example(s) of Type III reactions?

A. Methyldopa-induced haemolytic anaemia.
B. Bagassosis.
C. Pigeon breeder's lung.
D. Dengue haemorrhagic shock.
E. Autoimmune thyrotoxicosis.

7.12 Which of the following is/are true concerning a Type IV reaction?

A. There may be tissue necrosis.
B. Clinical effects vary according to antibody location.
C. There may be caseation.
D. Thrombocytopenia is typical.
E. Antigen-specific T cells react with antigen and release lymphokines.

7.13 Which of the following is/are the result of Type IV reactions?

A. Elephantiasis in filariasis.
B. Granulomatous reactions in schistosomiasis.
C. Myocarditis in Chagas' disease.
D. The nephrotic syndrome in malaria.
E. Katayama fever (acute schistosomiasis).

7.14 Which of the following is/are true concerning leprosy?

A. A positive lepromin test typifies lepromatous leprosy.
B. When the lepromin test is read at 4 weeks, it is called the Fernandez reaction.
C. The immune response is solely cell mediated.
D. There is a 10% incidence of false positive Wasserman reactions (WR).
E. Lepromatous and tuberculoid forms of the disease are serologically distinct.

Answers overleaf

7.11 B, C, D

Bagassosis, due to dried sugar cane, and pigeon breeder's lung, due to bird droppings, are examples of Type III reactions. Methyldopa haemolytic anaemia is a Type II reaction. Autoimmune thyrotoxicosis is due to thyroid-stimulating antibodies. In the past this was classified separately as a Type V reaction, but is now, in general, viewed as a Type II reaction. There is tissue stimulation then destruction. Dengue haemorrhagic fever is probably due to the failure of preformed antibodies from a previous infection by a different strain to neutralise the virus completely. This leads to a Type III response.

7.12 A, C, E

In a Type IV reaction, antigen-specific T cells react with antigen and release lymphokines which activate accessory cells. Unlike the Arthus reaction, the time scale is 24–48 hours. Macroscopically there is erythema, induration and eventually tissue necrosis. Caseation is typical of a Type IV reaction due to tuberculosis. Thrombocytopenia is not typical, and antibody does not play a role.

7.13 A, B

The nephrotic syndrome and Katayama fever are probably Type III reactions. Myocarditis in Chagas' disease is probably the result of a Type II reaction. Elephantiasis in filariasis and granulomatous reactions in schistosomiasis are due to Type IV reactions.

7.14 D

The lepromin test cannot be used to diagnose leprosy but can be used to determine the host's immune response. Leprosy encompasses a spectrum of disease varying from the lepromatous form, with poor cell-mediated immunity and negative lepromin test, to the tuberculoid form, where cell-mediated immunity is stronger and the lepromin test positive. Lesions tend to be localised in this form. The sera from 90% of lepromatous patients have antibodies to the bacillus. There is a 10% false positive WR. The two forms cannot be distinguished serologically. When the lepromin test is read at 72 hours, it is called the Fernandez reaction; when read at 4 weeks, it is called the Mitsuda reaction.

7.15 Concerning erythema nodosum leprosum, which of the following is/are true?

  A. It is due to circulating immune complexes.
  B. It is associated with iritis.
  C. It is associated with albuminuria.
  D. It is associated with amyloidosis.
  E. It can be treated by thalidomide.

7.16 Penicillins can induce which of the following reactions?

  A. Type I.
  B. Type II.
  C. Type III.
  D. Type IV.
  E. Type V.

7.17 Concerning drug-induced lupus erythematosus, which of the following is/are true?

  A. It more commonly produces clinical symptoms than does systemic lupus erythematosus (SLE).
  B. Hydrallazine is the most frequent cause of clinical disease.
  C. ANF is usually positive.
  D. Antibody titres against double-stranded DNA are usually high.
  E. Renal involvement is common.

Answers overleaf

7.15 All true

Erythema nodosum leprosum occurs in the lepromatous and borderline lepromatous forms of leprosy. It is an immune complex disease and usually develops when most of the bacilli are dead. The complexes activate complement and cause acute inflammation at their site of deposition. This leads to arthritis, iritis, neuritis of local nerves, and nephritis leading to albuminuria. Erythema nodosum appear on the shins. Persistent cases can develop amyloidosis. Mild cases respond to bedrest and aspirin. Moderate cases respond to clofazimine and steroids. Thalidomide can be used in the very severe case.

7.16 A, B, C, D

Penicillins can cause anaphylaxis (Type I), haemolytic anaemia (Type II), nephritis (Type III) and contact hypersensitivity (Type IV) reactions. Type V refers to autoimmune thyrotoxicosis and cannot be produced by penicillin (see question 7.11).

7.17 C

This disorder rarely produces clinical symptoms, but when these do occur they are most likely to be due to procainamide. Clinically the features are very similar to those of SLE, but renal and neural involvement is rare. ANF is usually positive with low levels of antibody to double-stranded DNA. Hydrallazine-induced lupus is associated with HLA-Dr 4, slow acetylators and antibodies to single-stranded DNA.

8. PRIMARY IMMUNODEFICIENCY STATES

8.1 Primary antibody deficiency is characterised by which of the following?

- **A.** Recurrent infections in the neonate.
- **B.** Chronic sinopulmonary disease.
- **C.** Chronic fungal infections.
- **D.** Poor resistance to chickenpox, mumps and measles.
- **E.** *Giardia lamblia* infections.

8.2 Concerning X-linked agammaglobulinaemia (Bruton's disease), which of the following is/are true?

- **A.** Immunoglobulins are usually undetectable.
- **B.** The thymus appears normal.
- **C.** Lymphopenia is common.
- **D.** One-third of patients have arthritis.
- **E.** There is an increased incidence of autoimmune disorders and lymphoreticular malignancies.

8.3 Which of the following is/are true concerning selective IgA deficiency?

- **A.** It is incompatible with good health.
- **B.** It is best treated with parenteral immune serum globulin which contains IgA.
- **C.** It is the commonest primary immunodeficiency disorder.
- **D.** It is due to a specific defect in the J component of IgA.
- **E.** It usually takes the form of low secretory IgA but normal serum IgA levels.

Answers overleaf

8.1 B, E

Maternal IgG acquired transplacentally generally protects the neonate with primary antibody deficiency. Hence infections usually start at 6–12 months of age; occasionally they are delayed until adolescence. Typical organisms include extracellular pyogenic bacteria and *Giardia lamblia*. Resistance to viruses is generally good except for enteroviruses and vaccinia. Systemic infections can be prevented by immune serum globulin injections, but there is no effective means of replacing IgA at the mucosal surfaces and many patients develop severe sinopulmonary disease.

8.2 B, D, E

Agammaglobulinaemia is a misnomer because usually a small amount of immunoglobulin is detectable. Lymphopenia is uncommon and the percentage of T cells is normal or elevated. Up to 6% of patients develop lymphoreticular malignancy and there is an increased incidence of autoimmune disorders. One-third of patients develop arthritis.

8.3 C

This is the commonest primary immunodeficiency disorder. Levels of secretory and serum IgA are very low, while other immunoglobulins are normal or elevated. It is occasionally seen in healthy individuals but is often associated with respiratory, gastrointestinal and urogenital infections. The basic defect is unknown. The only treatment is vigorous antimicrobial therapy when indicated. Parenteral immunoglobulin replacement fails to replace secretory IgA and carries the risk of anaphylaxis.

Primary Immunodeficiency States

8.4 Selective IgA deficiency is associated with which of the following?

A. Atopic diseases.
B. Autoimmune phenomena.
C. A sprue-like syndrome.
D. Anaphylactic reactions to blood products.
E. Serum antibodies against IgA.

8.5 Congenital cellular immunodeficiency is characterised by which of the following?

A. Autoimmune phenomena.
B. Growth retardation.
C. Atopic reactions.
D. Susceptibility to graft-versus-host disease.
E. A high incidence of malignancy.

8.6 Infections associated with congenital cellular immunodeficiency include which of the following?

A. Viruses.
B. Pyogenic bacteria.
C. Fungi.
D. *Pneumocystis carinii.*
E. *Strongyloides stercoralis.*

8.7 Which of the following occur(s) in di George's syndrome?

A. Maldevelopment of the third and fourth pharyngeal pouches.
B. Hypoplasia of the parathyroid glands.
C. Hypercalcaemia.
D. An association with cardiovascular abnormalities.
E. Strong evidence of inheritance.

Answers overleaf

Primary Immunodeficiency States
8.4 All true

As well as inhibiting entry of microbes via mucosal surfaces, secretory IgA also probably prevents adsorption of foreign antigens. Hence IgA deficiency is associated with antibodies and allergies to foods such as cow's milk. A sprue-like syndrome may develop which sometimes responds to a gluten-free diet. Autoantibodies are also common. Serum antibodies to IgA may be present in 44% of patients. Anaphylactic reactions may follow administration of blood products, and immune serum globulin containing IgA is contraindicated.

8.5 B, D, E

Graft-versus-host reactions may occur if the patient is given fresh blood or unmatched allogeneic bone marrow (see question 19.12). There is a high incidence of malignancies. Growth retardation occurs. Infections tend to be more difficult to treat than those occurring in antibody deficiency disorders because they are often due to fungi, viruses and atypical mycobacteria rather than bacteria.

8.6 A, C, D, E

T lymphocytes are important in defence against intracellular bacteria such as mycobacteria and *Listeria monocytogenes*. Neutrophils are important against pyogenic bacteria. T-cell impairment also predisposes to viral infection by measles and herpes. Other organisms typically infecting T-cell-deficient individuals include fungi (*Candida albicans, Cryptococcus neoformans, Aspergillus* species, *Histoplasma capsulatum*), protozoa (*Pneumocystis carinii, Toxoplasma gondii*), and helminths (*Strongyloides stercoralis*).

8.7 A, B, D

Maldevelopment of these pharyngeal pouches causes hypoplasia or aplasia of the thymus (hence cellular immunodeficiency) and parathyroids (hence hypocalcaemia). Other structures developing at the same age may be affected, causing, for example, congenital cardiovascular anomalies, oesophageal atresia, low-set notched ears and an antimongoloid slant to the eyes. There is little evidence of inheritance.

8.8 Duncan's syndrome is characterised by which of the following?

A. An impaired immune response to Epstein–Barr virus (EBV).
B. Uncontrolled T-cell proliferation.
C. Autosomal recessive inheritance.
D. Hypo- or dysgammaglobulinaemia.
E. Fatal lymphoproliferative disease.

8.9 Severe combined immunodeficiency (SCID) is associated with which of the following?

A. Deficiency of antibody, T cells and granulocytes.
B. Autosomal recessive inheritance.
C. X-linked recessive inheritance.
D. Adenosine deaminase deficiency.
E. Skeletal abnormalities.

8.10 Which of the following significantly increase(s) survival in SCID?

A. Thymus transplants.
B. Bone marrow transplants.
C. Parenteral immune serum globulins.
D. Prophylactic antibiotics.
E. Gnotobiotic isolation.

8.11 Wiskott–Aldrich syndrome is characterised by which of the following?

A. Eczema.
B. Megakaryocytic thrombocytopenic purpura.
C. Decreased synthesis of immunoglobulins.
D. Increased catabolism of immunoglobulins.
E. Aplastic thymus.

Answers overleaf

8.8 A, E

This is an X-linked recessive disorder named after the kindred in which it was first described. These individuals fail to produce an adequate antibody or T-cell response to EBV-induced B-cell proliferation. Uncontrolled B-cell proliferation may follow in association with lymphoreticular malignancies.

8.9 B, C, D, E

In SCID, congenital deficiency of antibody and T lymphocytes (but not granulocytes) predisposes to infections and graft-versus-host reactions. The autosomal recessive form is sometimes associated with absence of a purine salvage pathway enzyme, adenosine deaminase, and the presence of rib-cage abnormalities. The X-linked recessive SCID is not associated with enzyme or skeletal abnormalities.

8.10 B, E

Death usually occurs within the first year of life due to infection so that germ-free (gnotobiotic) isolation could increase survival. Bone marrow transplants from HLA-D compatible donors have been successful. Prophylactic antibiotics merely encourage colonisation with resistant organisms. Thymus transplants may be of value in di George's syndrome but not in SCID. Attempts at enzyme replacement have met with some immunological and clinical improvement in patients with adenosine deaminase deficiency.

8.11 A, B, D

This X-linked recessive syndrome is characterised clinically by the triad of eczema, thrombocytopenic purpura and increased susceptibility to infections. The rates of synthesis and catabolism of immunoglobulins are raised, resulting in very variable immuno-globulin levels.

8.12 Wiskott–Aldrich syndrome is associated with which of the following?

A. Antiplatelet antibodies.
B. Impaired humoral immunity to polysaccharide antigens.
C. Impaired cellular immunity and cutaneous anergy.
D. Autoimmune disorders.
E. Malignancies.

8.13 Typical clinical features of ataxia telangiectasia include which of the following?

A. Dermatitis.
B. Cerebellar ataxia.
C. Telangiectasia developing in the late teens.
D. Recurrent sinopulmonary infections.
E. Insulin-resistant diabetes.

8.14 Ataxia telangiectasia is associated with which of the following?

A. Low levels of alpha-fetoprotein.
B. Increased sensitivity of cells to ionising radiation.
C. Defective DNA repair.
D. Graft-versus-host disease.
E. Selective absence of IgM.

8.15 Chronic granulomatous disease is characterised by which of the following?

A. Hypogammaglobulinaemia.
B. Impaired delayed hypersensitivity.
C. Neutropenia.
D. Infections with *Staphylococcus aureus*.
E. A positive nitroblue tetrazolium (NBT) dye test.

Answers overleaf

8.12 B, C, E

The thrombocytopenia appears to be due to an intrinsic platelet abnormality. The survival time of homologous, but not autologous, platelets is normal. Impaired antibody response to polysaccharides is the earliest evidence of deficiency and infections occur due to bacteria with polysaccharide capsules (e.g. *Streptococcus pneumoniae*). Later, cellular immunity declines and infections due to *Pneumocystis carinii* and herpes viruses follow. Death usually occurs before adulthood, due to bleeding, infections, or malignancy (12%).

8.13 B, D, E

The cerebellar ataxia and oculocutaneous telangiectasia usually begin in the young child. There is an increased susceptibility to bacterial infections, especially sinopulmonary, and an increased incidence of diabetes mellitus. Inheritance appears to be autosomal recessive.

8.14 B, C

Cells from such patients have increased sensitivity to ionising irradiation, defective DNA repair and frequent chromosomal abnormalities. There is a high incidence of malignancies. Elevated alpha-fetoprotein has been noted. Cellular immunity is impaired but not absent. Selective absence of IgA is common (50–80%); IgE is usually low; IgG is low in 5–10%; IgM levels are generally normal.

8.15 D, E

The commonest variant is an X-linked disorder occurring usually in children. The defect lies in the inability of the neutrophil to kill certain micro-organisms after ingestion. Neutrophil number, morphology, chemotaxis and phagocytosis are normal. In the NBT dye test, the yellow dye is added to plasma and then these complexes are phagocytosed by neutrophils. Normally the complexes appear blue on microscopy due to reduction by lysosomal enzymes, but in chronic granulomatous disease this does not occur. Here, the complexes remain yellow and this is a positive test. Staphylococcal, enteric bacilli and fungal infections predominate.

8.16 Chronic mucocutaneous candidiasis has been associated with which of the following?

A. Specific immunological defects to *Candida* antigens.
B. No detectable immunological abnormality.
C. Bruton's X-linked agammaglobulinaemia.
D. Pregnancy.
E. Hypoparathyroidism.

8.17 A hypoplastic thymus is found in which of the following?

A. Multiple sclerosis.
B. Severe combined immunodeficiency (SCID).
C. Ataxia telangiectasia.
D. Wiskott–Aldrich syndrome.
E. Myasthenia gravis.

8.18 Concerning hereditary angioedema, which of the following is/are true?

A. C1 esterase inhibitor may be absent.
B. C1 esterase inhibitor may be present but inactive.
C. Abdominal pain may mimic an acute abdomen.
D. An analogous acquired form is associated with lymphoproliferative disorders.
E. Inheritance is autosomal recessive.

8.19 Complement deficiencies are associated with which of the following?

A. Chediak–Higashi syndrome.
B. Variable hypogammaglobulinaemia.
C. Susceptibility to bacterial infections.
D. Systemic lupus erythematosus (SLE).
E. Disseminated gonococcal sepsis.

Answers overleaf

8.16 A, B, E

This clinical syndrome probably has multiple causes. Sometimes it is associated with endocrine disorders or it may be part of a generalised cellular immunodeficiency (e.g. di George's syndrome) in which case *Candida albicans* is one of a number of opportunistic infections. In some cases the patient is only unresponsive to *Candida* antigens. However, many cases show no demonstrable immunological abnormality.

8.17 B, C

Myasthenia gravis is associated with thymomas. The thymus is normal in multiple sclerosis and in the Wiskott–Aldrich syndrome.

8.18 A, B, C, D

The inherited form of the disorder is autosomal dominant. It is characterised by episodes of oedema due to lack of or inactive C1 esterase inhibitor. Acquired C1 esterase deficiency is associated with low C4, C1 and C1q, rectal adenocarcinoma and lymphoproliferative disorders. Gastrointestinal oedema may cause abdominal pain.

8.19 C, D, E

C2 deficiency occurs in 1 in 200 patients with SLE compared with 1 in 10 000 of the general population. Deficiency of early complement components is associated with defective antigen clearance and bacterial infections. Deficiency of late components (C5–C8) is associated with recurrent meningococcal meningitis and disseminated gonococcal sepsis.

9. THE IMMUNOCOMPROMISED HOST

9.1 Concerning disseminated candidiasis, which of the following is/are true?

A. *Candida albicans* septicaemia is associated with neutropenia.
B. *Candida parapsilosis* septicaemia is associated with total parenteral feeding.
C. Local mucocutaneous candidiasis is associated with neutrophil defects.
D. Defective myeloperoxidase activity in neutrophils predisposes to invasive candidiasis.
E. Dissemination is indicated by a single positive blood culture.

9.2 Candidal oesophagitis is associated with which of the following?

A. Leukaemia.
B. Neutropenia.
C. Steroid therapy.
D. Alcoholism.
E. Lymphoma.

9.3 Ecthyma gangrenosa is associated with which of the following?

A. Gonococcal septicaemia.
B. Pneumococcal septicaemia.
C. *Pseudomonas* septicaemia.
D. Meningococcal septicaemia.
E. *Aeromonas* septicaemia.

Answers overleaf

The Immunocompromised Host

9.1 A, B, D

Candida albicans is the commonest cause of disseminated candidiasis. Local mucocutaneous forms are due either to inherited or to steroid-induced T-cell defects. Systemic forms are associated with neutropenia or defective neutrophils, as in myeloperoxidase deficiency. A single positive blood culture can be due to transient fungaemia after, for example, removal of a colonised catheter. *Candida parapsilosis* septicaemia is associated with total parenteral feeding.

9.2 All true

All the above can predispose to candidal oesophagitis.

9.3 C, E

Ecthyma gangrenosa is a vasculitic skin lesion with a black necrotic centre and raised erythematous border. It is associated with *Pseudomonas* and *Aeromonas* septicaemia. It may be a pointer to these infections in immunocompromised patients. The organisms can usually be isolated on blood culture.

9.4 An ecthyma gangrenosa-like lesion is associated with disseminated forms of which of the following conditions?

    A. Histoplasmosis.
    B. Mucormycosis.
    C. Candidiasis.
    D. Aspergillosis.
    E. Blastomycosis.

9.5 Which of the following predispose(s) to dissemination of coccidioidomycosis in immunocompromised patients?

    A. Lymphocytopenia.
    B. Neutropenia.
    C. Skin test positivity to spherulin.
    D. Possession of blood group B.
    E. Cytoxic therapy.

9.6 Which of the following predispose(s) to dissemination in aspergillosis?

    A. Defects in immunoglobulin production.
    B. Defects in late complement components.
    C. Neutropenia.
    D. Primary cytomegalovirus (CMV) infection.
    E. Renal transplantation.

9.7 Splenectomy leads to which of the following?

    A. Decreased levels of serum IgM.
    B. Increased levels of properdin.
    C. Enhanced susceptibility to infection by encapsulated bacteria.
    D. Decreased levels of tuftsin.
    E. Increased levels of serum IgA.

Answers overleaf

9.4 B, D

Disseminated mucormycosis and aspergillosis produce an ecthyma gangrenosa-like lesion. This differs from ecthyma gangrenosa in that one can isolate fungus from a biopsy of the lesion.

9.5 A, D, E

Predisposition to dissemination is caused by lymphocytopenia, cytotoxic therapy and possession of blood group B. A positive skin test to spherulin means that the immune response is good and dissemination unlikely.

9.6 C, D, E

Primary CMV infection rather than secondary reactivation seems to be associated with dissemination of *Aspergillus*. Neutropenia occurs in both CMV and disseminated *Aspergillus* infections. Renal transplants are predisposed to CMV (infection or reactivation) and disseminated aspergillosis.

9.7 A, C, D

Following splenectomy, the levels of IgM, properdin and tuftsin are decreased. The low level of properdin is probably responsible for the impairment of the alternate pathway of complement. Because of the enhanced susceptibility to encapsulated bacteria, immunisation with polyvalent pneumococcal vaccine is desirable. Tuftsin is a phagocytosis-promoting peptide.

9.8 A patient with a lymphoma develops meningitis, which of the following is/are the likeliest cause(s).

A. If bacterial, *Listeria monocytogenes*.
B. If fungal, *Cryptococcus neoformans*.
C. If protozoal, trichomonads.
D. If viral, Coxsackie B.
E. If post-splenectomy, *Staphylococcus aureus*.

9.9 A patient who has had an organ transplant and systemic steroid immunosuppression develops a brain abscess. Which of the following is/are the likeliest cause(s)?

A. If bacterial, *Nocardia asteroides*.
B. If fungal, *Cryptococcus neoformans*.
C. If parasitic, *Toxoplasma gondii*.
D. If viral, a papovavirus.
E. If post-splenectomy, *Legionella pneumophilia*.

9.10 In patients with a total peripheral white count of less than $1000/mm^3$, which of the following is/are true?

A. The likeliest cause of bacterial meningitis is enteric bacilli.
B. The likeliest cause of bacterial cerebral abscess is enteric bacilli.
C. The likeliest cause of a fungal cerebral abscess is *Candida* species.
D. The likeliest cause of fungal meningitis is *Aspergillus* species.
E. Meningoencephalitis can be caused by the zygomycoses.

9.11 Concerning *Pneumocystis* pneumonia, which of the following is/are true?

A. Haemoptysis occurs in 90% of cases.
B. There is typically a diffuse bilateral alveolar infiltrate.
C. Pleural effusion occurs in about 5% of cases.
D. The development of drug resistance has lead to the use of high-dose septrin rather than pentamidine for treatment.
E. The diagnosis can be made serologically.

Answers overleaf

9.8 A, B

In lymphomas, depression of the T-lymphocyte response predisposes to viral infections of the varicella zoster–herpes simplex group, and this is the commonest cause of viral meningitis. The commonest parasitic causes of meningitis are *Toxoplasma gondii* (protozoan) and *Strongyloides stercoralis* (helminth). The commonest bacterial cause in patients with lymphoma is *Listeria monocytogenes*. Post-splenectomy, encapsulated bacteria are commoner, in particular *Streptococcus pneumoniae, Haemophilus influenzae* and *Neisseria meningitidis*. The commonest fungal cause of meningitis in patients with lymphoma is *Cryptococcus neoformans*. The likeliest causes of meningitis in organ transplant recipients are the same.

9.9 A, B, C, D

Patients with lymphoma or organ transplant recipients on systemic steroids have depressed T-lymphocyte and macrophage function. The likeliest causes of brain abscesses are the same for both groups of patients. *Nocardia asteroides* is the likeliest bacterial cause of a brain abscess in the two groups. *Legionella pneumophilia* does not cause brain abscesses. *Papovaviridae* are the likeliest viral cause of a brain abscess.

9.10 A, B, E

The likeliest bacterial cause of meningitis or a cerebral abscess in leucopenic patients is an enteric Gram-negative rod. Fungal meningitis is most commonly due to a *Candida* species, whereas a cerebral abscess is most likely to be due to an *Aspergillus* species. Meningoencephalitis is occasionally caused by one of the zygomycoses.

9.11 B, C, E

Haemoptysis is relatively unusual in *Pneumocystis* pneumonia. The chest x-ray characteristically shows a bilateral diffuse alveolar infiltrate. Pleural effusions occur in about 5% of cases. Septrin is the preferred drug treatment because it is less toxic than pentamidine. Diagnosis is made histologically or serologically, by indirect immunofluorescence. The absence of antibody does not exclude the possibility of infection.

9.12 Patients with diabetes mellitus are more prone to develop which of the following infections?

   A. Mucormycosis.
   B. Candidiasis.
   C. Tuberculosis.
   D. Gas gangrene.
   E. Staphylococcal carbuncles.

9.13 Eczema herpeticum (Kaposi's varicelliform eruption) is associated with which of the following?

   A. Darrier's disease.
   B. Atopic eczema.
   C. Wiskott–Aldrich syndrome.
   D. Lymphoreticular malignancies of the skin.
   E. Pemphigus.

9.14 Concerning cytomegalovirus (CMV) infections in renal transplant recipients, which of the following is/are true?

   A. Symptoms usually develop within 1 month of transplantation.
   B. The time of onset of symptoms differs between primary infection and reactivation of a latent infection.
   C. Symptoms are more severe in recipients of cadaveric kidneys than in those receiving kidneys from live donors.
   D. Treatment includes increasing the dosage of immunosuppressant therapy.
   E. Death is usually due to superinfection with bacteria or protozoa.

Answers overleaf

9.12 All true

These five diseases all occur more frequently and with increased morbidity in diabetes. Tuberculosis was a particularly common cause of death before insulin became available.

9.13 All True

Eczema herpeticum is a widespread cutaneous dissemination of herpes simplex. The commonest skin disease predisposing to eczema herpeticum is atopic eczema. Other rarer skin diseases predisposing to the condition are Darrier's disease and pemphigus, where the epidermal structure is disorganised. In the lymphoreticular malignancies the lesion lies in failure of the T lymphocytes to control the viral infection and, as well as eczema herpeticum, visceral dissemination may occur, carrying a mortality of 10–50%. In Wiskott–Aldrich syndrome, impaired cellular immunity later predisposes to herpes infections (see question 8.12).

9.14 C, E

The symptoms of CMV virtually always develop 1–4 months after transplantation, regardless of whether infection is primary or due to reactivation of the latent virus. Recipients of cadaveric kidneys receive more immunosuppressive therapy and therefore develop more severe infections than the recipients of kidneys from living donors. Immunosuppressants can be successfully reduced as part of the treatment of CMV occurring in transplant recipients because CMV is itself an immunosuppressant. Death is usually due to superinfection with bacteria or protozoa, particularly *Pneumocystis carinii*.

9.15 **Concerning hepatitis B infections in the immunocompromised host, which of the following is/are true?**

   A. Serology gives a false negative in 60% of cases.
   B. Liver biopsy is essential.
   C. Fulminant hepatitis is likely in patients with di George's syndrome.
   D. Mild hepatitis is likely in severe X-linked agammaglobulinaemia.
   E. Serum aminotransferase levels are usually normal or minimally elevated.

9.16 **Cytomegalovirus (CMV) infection in a renal transplant recipient may cause which of the following?**

   A. Thrombocytopenia.
   B. Leucopenia.
   C. Atypical lymphocytes in the peripheral blood smear.
   D. Abnormal liver function tests.
   E. Chorioretinitis.

9.17 **Depressed cellular immunity makes a patient more likely to develop pulmonary infection caused by which of the following organisms?**

   A. *Staphylococcus aureus.*
   B. *Pneumocystis carinii.*
   C. *Toxoplasma gondii.*
   D. *Strongyloides stercoralis.*
   E. Cytomegalovirus.

9.18 **In the immunocompromised host, cavitation is found in pneumonia caused by which of the following?**

   A. *Nocardia asteroides.*
   B. *Klebsiella pneumoniae.*
   C. *Pseudomonas aeruginosa.*
   D. Mucormycosis.
   E. *Streptococcus pneumoniae.*

Answers overleaf

9.15 E

As in normal individuals, hepatitis B infection in immuno-compromised patients is diagnosed serologically and not by liver biopsy. Inherited B-lymphocyte deficiencies such as severe X-linked agammaglobulinaemia are associated with severe hepatitis. In T-cell deficiencies, such as di George's syndrome, the hepatitis is usually mild. Immunocompromised patients show only a small rise in aminotransferase levels in response to infection.

9.16 All true

Leucopenia (often fewer than 1500/mm^3) and/or thrombocytopenia (fewer than 100 000/mm^3) occur almost as commonly as pneumonia in renal transplant recipients developing CMV. Atypical lymphocytes may be seen in the peripheral blood, and liver function tests may be abnormal. Chorioretinitis is a late complication occurring after about 6 months.

9.17 B, C, D, E

Depressed cellular immunity due to T-lymphocyte dysfunction generally predisposes to viral, fungal, mycobacterial and protozoal pneumonias. In contrast, B-lymphocyte deficiencies are associated with frequent infections with extracellular pyogenic bacteria such as *Staphylococcus aureus* and *Streptococcus pneumoniae*.

9.18 A, B, C, D

Cavitation suggests a necrotising infection such as that caused by *Nocardia asteroides,* Gram-negative bacilli (most commonly *Klebsiella pneumoniae* and *Pseudomonas aeruginosa)*, fungi (as in mucormycosis and aspergillosis), *Staphylococcus aureus* and tuberculosis.

9.19 **Which of the following statements is/are true concerning the acquired immunodeficiency syndrome (AIDS)?**

A. There is an increased incidence in Ashkanazi Jews.
B. A similar disease has been described in rhesus monkeys.
C. There can be a prodromal illness of lymphadenopathy, diarrhoea and weight loss.
D. It is commoner than expected in Haitians.
E. It is associated with Kaposi's sarcoma.

9.20 **Which of the following epidemiological facts is/are true concerning the acquired immunodeficiency syndrome?**

A. 10% of cases are homosexual.
B. 40% of cases are intravenous drug abusers.
C. 20% of cases have no obvious risk factor.
D. 30% of cases are haemophiliacs.
E. 30% of cases are female.

Answers overleaf

9.19 B, C, D, E

AIDS is a newly described syndrome which links an uncommon form of cancer, Kaposi's sarcoma, with a whole range of infections. Kaposi's sarcoma was, until the advent of AIDS, a slowly developing indolent tumour usually localised to the lower extremities. It was commoner in Ashkanazi Jews, especially elderly males in their seventh decade. The form found in association with AIDS attacks a much younger age group and does not have the same ethnic predisposition. It was first described in the United States. There is an increased incidence in Haitians. A prodromal illness with lymphadenopathy, diarrhoea and weight loss occurs in about 10% of cases. A similar disease has been described in rhesus monkeys.

9.20 All false

AIDS is associated with a 75% incidence of homosexuality and a 13% incidence of drug abuse. In 5% there is no obvious risk factor, and less than 1% of current cases are haemophiliacs. The incidence in women is about 6%.

The Immunocompromised Host

9.21 Which of the following infectious agents is/are commoner in the acquired immunodeficiency syndrome?

A. *Pneumocystis carinii.*
B. *Candida albicans.*
C. *Cryptococcus neoformans.*
D. *Mycobacterium avium-intracellulare.*
E. Genital warts.

9.22 Which of the following immunological abnormalities have been found in the acquired immunodeficiency syndrome?

A. Thrombocytopenic purpura.
B. An increased level of Natural Killer cells.
C. Elevated alpha-1 thymosin levels.
D. A reversed T helper : T suppressor ratio.
E. An increased incidence of systemic lupus erythematosus (SLE).
F. Hypergammaglobulinaemia.
G. Failure to make antibody in response to immunisation.
H. Lymphopenia.
I. Defective skin sensitivity to purified protein derivative (PPD).
J. Neutropenia.

Answers overleaf

9.21 All true

Other infectious agents associated with AIDS include *Entamoeba histolytica,* herpes simplex, cytomegalovirus and cryptosporidium.

9.22 A, C, D, E, F, G, H, I

AIDS is associated with a reversed T-helper to T-suppressor ratio and profound immunodeficiency. The normal ratio of T-helper to T-suppressor cells is about 1.8 but in AIDS it may be only 0.8. Natural Killer cells are diminished in number. There is lymphopenia and not neutropenia. There is an increased incidence of SLE, and thrombocytopenic purpura. Elevated levels of alpha-1 thymosin, a thymic hormone thought to be involved in T-cell maturation, are thought to represent a compensatory thymic response to T-helper depletion. Skin sensitivity to various antigens (e.g. PPD) is impaired. Paradoxically, although there is hypergammaglobulinaemia, there is failure to make antibody upon immunisation. The hypergammaglobulinaemia may be related to polyclonal B-cell activation following reactivation of latent Epstein–Barr virus.

10. CONNECTIVE TISSUE DISEASES

10.1 Systemic lupus erythematosus (SLE) is characterised by which of the following?

A. The formation of immune complexes.
B. Frequent skin and joint involvement.
C. A butterfly face rash with follicular plugging and scarring.
D. 'Wire loop' lesions and 'haematoxylin bodies' in the kidney.
E. 'Onion skin' thickening in the spleen.

10.2 Concerning SLE, which of the following is/are true?

A. Pulmonary involvement is generally the most important prognostic factor.
B. Libman–Sachs endocarditis is the commonest cardiac complication.
C. High complement levels indicate active renal disease.
D. Leucocytosis is usual.
E. Joint erosions are common.

10.3 Which of the following is/are true concerning the DNA binding test as used in the diagnosis of SLE?

A. It is based on the Farr technique.
B. It assays antibody to native (double-stranded) DNA.
C. It assays antibody to heat-denatured (single-stranded) DNA.
D. It is usually high in discoid LE.
E. It is the best laboratory test for monitoring renal disease activity.

Answers overleaf

10.1 All true

SLE is the classical example of immune complex disease in man. Deposits of immunoglobulin and complement appear 'lumpy' using immunofluorescence in renal, skin and vascular lesions. DNA antigens predominate. Skin and joint diseases are the most frequent complaints. A characteristic feature is the facial butterfly rash. Pathological changes in the skin include *f*ollicular plugging, *a*trophy, *t*elangiectasia, *e*rythema and *s*carring (FATES). 'Haematoxylin bodies' may be found within the glomerular capillary loops. They are the tissue counterpart of the LE cell. 'Wire loop' lesions may be seen in advanced cases. 'Onion skin' lesions in the spleen are due to concentric periarterial fibrosis.

10.2 All false

Renal, cardiac and central nervous system lesions are the most important prognostically. Involvement of the pericardium and, secondly, myocarditis are both commoner than the rare 'Libman–Sachs' sterile vegetations. Low complement levels correlate with active renal disease. Leucopenia, especially lymphopenia, is common and helps differentiate from other vasculitides. Arthralgia and synovitis occur in most patients but joint erosions are rare.

10.3 A, B

Anti-DNA antibodies reacting to native double-stranded DNA are highly specific to SLE, unlike those reacting to denatured single-stranded DNA. Using a technique based on the Farr assay, the patient's serum is added to radiolabelled DNA and the resulting DNA–anti-DNA complex precipitated with 50% saturated ammonium sulphate. The relative radioactivity of the supernatant and precipitate gives the 'DNA binding' value. It is positive in 80–100% of cases of SLE and rarely in chronic active hepatitis and Felty's syndrome. Most cases of drug-induced lupus and discoid LE give normal binding values. The test gives some indication of general disease activity but serial complement values give a better estimate of renal involvement.

10.4 Antibodies against which of the following nuclear and nucleolar components is/are characteristically found in SLE?

A. Single-stranded RNA.
B. Double-stranded RNA.
C. The ribonucleoprotein (RNP) component of 'extractable nuclear antigen' (ENA).
D. The Sm antigen component of ENA.
E. Nucleolar RNA.

10.5 Concerning antinuclear factors (ANF), which of the following is/are true?

A. They are detected by means of direct immunofluorescence.
B. A speckled pattern of immunofluorescence is associated with mixed connective tissue disease.
C. Antinuclear antibodies directed against granulocyte nuclei are occasionally found in rheumatoid arthritis.
D. Low titres are common and non-specific.
E. They are positive in up to 75% of SLE patients.

10.6 Features suggestive of Sjøgren's syndrome include which of the following?

A. Lymphocytic infiltration of the salivary glands.
B. Burning of the eyes.
C. Psychosis.
D. Ectopia lentis.
E. Alopecia.

10.7 Sjøgren's syndrome is associated with which of the following?

A. Renal tubular acidosis.
B. Hypogammaglobulinaemia.
C. Lymphoma.
D. Primary biliary cirrhosis.
E. Myasthenia gravis.

Answers overleaf

Connective Tissue Diseases

10.4 B, D

Human RNA is mainly single stranded. In SLE, antibody against double-stranded RNA (possibly viral) is detectable in about a third of cases. Unlike DNA binding, the titres do not reflect disease activity. Antibody against the ribonucleoprotein component of a group of nuclear proteins called 'extractable nuclear antigen' (ENA) is associated with mixed connective tissue disease. The Sm component of ENA is a saline-soluble, non-nucleic acid component. Antibody to Sm is highly specific for SLE. (Sm is named after a patient called Smith.) Nucleolar RNA antibodies are common in scleroderma.

10.5 B, C, D

ANF is usually detected by indirect immunofluorescence using human thyroid or rat liver as nuclear antigen. The unlabelled ANF in the patient's serum is then detected using a second fluorochrome-labelled conjugated antiserum. It is positive in 98% of SLE patients. Patterns of immunofluorescence may be of some diagnostic use in that a speckled pattern is associated with mixed connective tissue disease. Granulocyte-specific ANF may occur in rheumatoid arthritis. Low titres of ANF are common and not diagnostic.

10.6 A, B

In Sjøgren's syndrome, intense salivary gland infiltration by lymphocytes leads to their destruction and xerostomia (dry mouth). A similar mechanism causes keratoconjunctivitis sicca which presents as burning or grittiness of the eyes. This may progress to superficial corneal scarring and then keratitis filamentosa. Psychosis and alopecia are typical of SLE and not Sjøgren's syndrome. Sjøgren's syndrome and SLE may occur in the same patient. Ectopia lentis is displacement of the lens in the eye and is found in Marfan's syndrome.

10.7 A, C, D, E

Renal disorders associated with Sjøgren's syndrome involve the tubules rather than the glomeruli and renal tubular acidosis occurs in about a quarter of patients. The hypergammaglobulinaemia characteristic of the syndrome may be partly responsible. Associations include primary biliary cirrhosis, myasthenia gravis and lymphoproliferative disorders of varying degrees of malignancy. The last-mentioned may be due to irradiation of salivary glands in the past.

10.8 **Patients with rheumatoid arthritis who have a high titre of ANF are more likely to have or develop which of the following?**

    A. Keratoconjunctivitis sicca.
    B. Hepatomegaly.
    C. Hypersensitivity to penicillin.
    D. Xerostomia.
    E. Neutropenia.

10.9 **Concerning the ANF found in patients with rheumatoid arthritis, which of the following is/are true?**

    A. It is of the IgG class.
    B. It gives a speckled pattern of immunofluorescence.
    C. It is associated with high DNA-binding values.
    D. It is never associated with LE cells in rheumatoid patients.
    E. It is an indication for a Schirmer's test.

10.10 **Which of the following is/are true concerning rheumatoid factors (Rf), as measured by the latex agglutination test?**

    A. They are antibodies directed against the Fc portion of IgM-coated latex particles.
    B. They are of the IgG class.
    C. They are anticomplementary.
    D. They are associated with a worse prognosis than Rf-negative cases in rheumatoid arthritis.
    E. They are less specific than those measured by the sheep cell agglutination test.

10.11 **A positive Rf is associated with which of the following?**

    A. SLE.
    B. Scleroderma.
    C. Polyarteritis nodosa.
    D. Bacterial endocarditis.
    E. Sarcoidosis.

Answers overleaf

10.8 A, C, D, E

Patients with rheumatoid arthritis who have high ANF titres generally have more severe disease. They are more likely to develop Sjøgren's syndrome (keratoconjunctivitis sicca, xerostomia) and Felty's syndrome (splenomegaly, neutropenia), and are more likely to be hypersensitive to penicillin.

10.9 E

The ANF associated with rheumatoid arthritis differs from that occurring in SLE in that it is mainly IgM, not IgG, and it is not associated with high levels of anti-DNA antibodies. However, LE cells may be present. The ANF gives a homogeneous pattern of immunofluorescence. It is an indication for a Schirmer's tear test to screen for Sjøgren's syndrome.

10.10 C, D, E

Rheumatoid factors are directed against the Fc portion of human or animal IgG. Those detected by the commonly used agglutination tests are generally IgM. The latex agglutination test is more widely used than the sheep cell agglutination test and is more sensitive but less specific. Rf is anticomplementary (i.e. fixes complement) and may have other protective roles but whether its presence is beneficial or harmful overall is unknown. Rf-positive cases generally have a worse prognosis.

10.11 A, B, D, E

As well as with rheumatoid arthritis and Sjøgren's syndrome, a positive Rf is associated with SLE, scleroderma, paraproteinaemia, sarcoidosis, chronic liver disease and various chronic infections such as syphilis and bacterial endocarditis. Relatives of rheumatoid patients and the elderly are also more likely to be Rf positive.

10.12 A 24-year-old woman gave a 2-year history of mild non-erosive
arthritis and severe depression which first began when she
started taking oral contraceptives. She was hypersensitive to
penicillin. On examination she was found to have a pericardial
friction rub and proteinuria (greater than 3.5 g). Which of the
following is the likeliest diagnosis?

A. Rheumatoid arthritis.
B. Rheumatic fever.
C. Mixed connective tissue disease.
D. SLE.
E. Polyarteritis nodosa.

10.13 Which of the following disorders is/are commoner in women
than men and commoner in Negroes than Caucasians?

A. Rheumatoid arthritis.
B. SLE.
C. Scleroderma.
D. Polymyositis.
E. Relapsing polychondritis.

10.14 Which of the following joints is/are commonly clinically affected
in seropositive rheumatoid arthritis?

A. The wrists.
B. The distal interphalangeal joints.
C. The sacroiliac joints.
D. The atlanto-axial joint.
E. The metatarsophalangeal joints.

10.15 Which of the following changes is/are typical of a rheumatoid
joint?

A. Villous hypertrophy.
B. Plasma cell and lymphocyte infiltration of the synovium.
C. Pannus formation.
D. High levels of complement in the synovial fluid.
E. Bone fusion.

Answers overleaf

10.12 D

The non-erosive arthritis makes rheumatoid arthritis very unlikely. The renal involvement makes mixed connective tissue disease relatively unlikely. The patient's age, sex, hypersensitivity to penicillin, pericardial, renal, and nervous involvement make SLE the likeliest diagnosis. Rheumatic fever and polyarteritis nodosa will only explain some of the features.

10.13 B, C

In SLE and Sjøgren's syndrome, the female:male ratio is 9:1. In rheumatoid arthritis and scleroderma the ratio is about 3:1. Polymyositis and relapsing polychondritis are commoner in men than women. SLE and scleroderma are commoner in Negroes.

10.14 A, D, E

The wrists are the commonest joints to be affected in rheumatoid arthritis and provide early radiological evidence of disease. Involvement of the metatarsophalangeal joints may also present early. Atlanto-axial joint involvement may lead to subluxation and pressure on the spinal cord which may present suddenly as spinal cord compression. Both distal interphalangeal joint involvement and sacroiliitis are rare in seropositive rheumatoid. The former may be due to psoriasis.

10.15 A, B, C

Initially there is vascular congestion and dilatation associated with oedema and polymorph infiltration of the synovium. The synovium hypertrophies, producing villi, and becomes infiltrated with plasma cells and lymphocytes which aggregate as follicles. A 'pannus' of granulation tissue consisting of fibroblasts, blood vessels and inflammatory cells spreads over and erodes into the cartilage and bone. Synovial fluid complement levels tend to be low, unlike in the seronegative arthritidies in which they are high. Serum complement levels are normal or high in rheumatoid arthritis. Bone fusion is a feature of Still's disease, but rare in rheumatoid arthritis.

10.16 **Which of the following is the commonest ocular manifestation of rheumatoid arthritis?**

  A. Iritis.
  B. Keratoconjunctivitis sicca.
  C. Uveitis.
  D. Scleritis.
  E. Scleromalacia perforans.

10.17 **Concerning Still's disease, which of the following is/are true?**

  A. Presentation may be acute with fever, rash, leucocytosis and pericarditis.
  B. Iritis is most likely to occur in children with widespread arthritis.
  C. A positive ANF is associated with increased risk of developing iritis.
  D. Amyloidosis occurs in 2–6% of patients.
  E. A positive Rf is of no prognostic value.

10.18 **Which of the following is/are found in rheumatoid nodules?**

  A. Giant cells.
  B. Epithelioid cells.
  C. Eosinophils.
  D. Monocytes.
  E. Plasma cells.

10.19 **Which of the following is/are well-recognised site(s) for rheumatoid nodules?**

  A. The elbow.
  B. The scalp.
  C. The popliteal fossa.
  D. The lung.
  E. Along the course of tendons.

Answers overleaf

10.16 B

Iritis is a complication of Still's disease and not rheumatoid arthritis. Keratoconjunctivitis sicca is the commonest ocular manifestation of rheumatoid arthritis. Episcleritis, scleritis, uveitis and scleromalacia perforans (development of a rheumatoid nodule in the sclera) are relatively rare complications. Chloroquine may cause a dose-related retinopathy.

10.17 A, C, D

Still's disease (juvenile rheumatoid arthritis) may present acutely with systemic disease or more insidiously with polyarticular or monoarticular involvement. Iritis (in 5–20%) and amyloidosis (2–6%) are two important complications. The former most frequently develops in children with monoarthritis or oligoarthritis, especially those with a positive ANF test. Amyloidosis tends to occur in those with progressive polyarticular disease. IgM rheumatoid factor is associated with an increased risk of progression to adult-like rheumatoid arthritis.

10.18 D, E

Rheumatoid nodules consist of three zones: an inner necrotic zone, surrounded by a palisade of mononuclear cells (including histiocytes and monocytes) and an outer layer of plasma cells, lymphocytes and fibroblasts. Evidence of arteritis may also be present.

10.19 A, B, D, E

Rheumatoid nodules are most commonly subcutaneous and occur at pressure points, such as the elbows, and along tendons and in the scalp. Flexor surfaces, such as the popliteal fossa, are spared. However, they can occur in intradermal, subperiosteal or visceral sites, including the mitral and aortic valves and the lung.

10.20 **Cases of 'seronegative' rheumatoid athritis are less likely than 'seropositive' cases to have which of the following?**

A. Severe joint disease.
B. Rheumatoid nodules.
C. Vasculitis.
D. Sjøgren's syndrome.
E. IgG Rf.

10.21 **Peripheral neuropathy is frequent in which of the following?**

A. Scleroderma.
B. Rheumatoid arthritis.
C. Polymyositis.
D. Polyarteritis nodosa.
E. SLE.

10.22 **Pericarditis is a recognised complication of which of the following?**

A. Polymyositis.
B. SLE
C. Mixed connective tissue disease.
D. Polyarteritis nodosa.
E. Rheumatoid arthritis.

10.23 **Pleurisy is a common manifestation of which of the following?**

A. Polyarteritis nodosa.
B. Relapsing polychondritis.
C. Rheumatoid arthritis.
D. SLE.
E. Polymyositis.

Answers overleaf

10.20 A, B, C, D

'Seronegative' cases lack IgM Rf but usually have IgG Rf. They are much less likely to develop nodules, vasculitis, neuropathy, Felty's or Sjøgren's syndrome. Patients with high Rf IgM levels are the most likely to develop severe joint disease.

10.21 B, D

Peripheral neuropathy is rare in SLE but is relatively common in rheumatoid arthritis and polyarteritis nodosa. In rheumatoid arthritis the carpal tunnel syndrome is probably the commonest form. A symmetrical, usually sensory, peripheral neuropathy has also been described. In polyarteritis nodosa, the peripheral neuropathy is predominantly motor, usually asymmetrical and affects mainly the legs. Mononeuritis multiplex may occur in rheumatoid arthritis and polyarteritis nodosa due to arteritis of the vasa nervorum.

10.22 B, D, E

Pericarditis is the most frequent cardiac complication in SLE and rheumatoid arthritis. It occurs secondary to coronary arteritis and myocardial infarction in polyarteritis nodosa. A fibrotic form of pericarditis occurs in scleroderma.

10.23 C, D

SLE characteristically affects serosal surfaces causing pericarditis, peritonitis and pleurisy—one of the commonest manifestations of SLE. Pleurisy may be the presenting complaint in rheumatoid arthritis. Pulmonary fibrosis may also occur in SLE and rheumatoid arthritis. Pleurisy is rare in classical polyarteritis nodosa.

Connective Tissue Diseases

10.24 Livedo reticularis is a feature of which of the following?

A. Polymyositis.
B. Amantadine treatment of Parkinson's disease.
C. Polyarteritis nodosa.
D. SLE.
E. Scleroderma.

10.25 A 50-year-old woman presents with severe Raynaud's phenomenon. Which of the following is the likeliest cause?

A. Cryoglobulinaemia.
B. Cervical rib.
C. Sjøgren's syndrome.
D. SLE.
E. Scleroderma.

10.26 Pulmonary involvement in scleroderma is characterised by which of the following?

A. Apical fibrosis.
B. Finger clubbing.
C. Development of pulmonary hypertension.
D. Increased incidence of alveolar or bronchiolar carcinoma.
E. Bronchial calcification.

10.27 Dermatological features of scleroderma include which of the following?

A. Calcification.
B. Pigmentation.
C. Vitiligo.
D. Telangiectasia.
E. Periungal infarcts.

Answers overleaf

10.24 C, D

Livedo reticularis is a blotchy bluish cutaneous manifestation of vasculitis and may be seen in SLE and polyarteritis nodosa. Occasionally it occurs in apparently healthy persons. When it occurs following amantadine treatment in Parkinson's disease, it is not serious and can be ignored. If pronounced erythematous oedema of the ankles occurs, amantadine should be discontinued.

10.25 E

All the above may cause Raynaud's phenomenon but severe Raynaud's phenomenon in this age group is most likely to be due to scleroderma. The Raynaud's may precede the scleroderma by many months. Mixed connective tissue disease is another important cause of Raynaud's phenomenon and should be excluded.

10.26 C, D

The pulmonary fibrosis occurs mainly in the lower lobes, and cystic changes in the periphery in some patients give a 'honeycomb lung'. Clubbing is not a feature. It is not associated with bronchial calcification though the pleura may become thickened and calcified. Chest infections are common. Pulmonary hypertension is a frequent complication and cause of death. Alveolar cell or bronchiolar carcinoma may develop as a relatively rare complication of the fibrosis.

10.27 A, B, C, D

Calcification most commonly occurs at the finger-tips but may be widespread (Thibierge–Weissenbach syndrome). Telangiectasia usually occurs on the cheeks and around the lips but is occasionally widespread. Pigmentation or, especially in Negroes, vitiligo may occur. The tightness of the skin around the fingers, nose and mouth is characteristic. Periungal infarcts are a manifestation of the vasculitis found in rheumatoid arthritis. Cutaneous manifestations may be memorised as 'CRST' (calcinosis, Raynaud's phenomenon, sclerodactyly and telangiectasia).

10.28 Which of the following is/are NOT associated with scleroderma?

   A. Anti-RNA antibodies.
   B. Dysphagia.
   C. Polyarthritis.
   D. Cardiac conduction defects.
   E. Psychosis.

10.29 Which of the following is/are true concerning LE cells?

   A. They are due to the presence of circulating IgG which reacts with nuclear DNA histone.
   B. They are commoner in SLE than in drug-induced lupus erythematosus.
   C. They are commoner in SLE than in discoid lupus erythematosus (DLE).
   D. They occur in rheumatoid-associated Sjøgren's syndrome.
   E. They are common in all connective tissue disorders.

Answers overleaf

10.28 E

Anti-RNA antibodies, probably against the uracil component of RNA, have been described in scleroderma. Oesophageal involvement is usual and leads to dysphagia and reflux oesophagitis. Polyarthritis occurs in about a quarter of patients. Fibrosis of the myocardium and pericardium may occur, the former leading to conduction defects. Neural involvement does not occur in scleroderma.

10.29 A, C, D

The IgG responsible for LE cells reacts with histone in the nuclei of a variety of tissues. LE cells are found in the blood of 80% of patients with either SLE or drug-induced lupus erythematosus. Only 20% of cases of DLE have LE cells. They are rare in other disorders with the exception of rheumatoid-associated Sjøgren's syndrome and chronic active hepatitis.

11. ORGAN-SPECIFIC IMMUNITY

I: Dermatology

11.1 Atopic dermatitis is characterised by which of the following?

  A. Onset during adolescence.
  B. Pruritus.
  C. Flexural lichenification in infancy.
  D. Low serum IgE levels.
  E. Increased susceptibility to viral infections.

11.2 Atopic dermatitis is associated with which of the following?

  A. Asthma.
  B. Allergic rhinitis.
  C. White dermographism.
  D. Cataracts.
  E. Phenylketonuria.

11.3 Concerning urticaria, which of the following is/are true?

  A. Oedema is always confined to the skin.
  B. Type I hypersensitivity is sometimes involved.
  C. It may be the sole manifestation of hereditary angioedema.
  D. It may be induced by heat or cold.
  E. In 75% of cases the cause is known.

Answers overleaf

11.1 B, E

Atopic dermatitis usually begins at 3–6 months of age. There is a strong hereditary predisposition. The condition is characterised by pruritus and lichenification. In infancy the forehead, cheeks and extensor surfaces are usually involved. Later in life the distribution alters to involve flexural surfaces, mainly popliteal and antecubital. Atopic dermatitis appears to be a cutaneous form of Type I hypersensitivity. Serum IgE levels are high. T-cell function appears to be depressed leading to increased susceptibility to widespread viral infections such as vaccinia and herpes simplex.

11.2 All true

Atopic dermatitis is associated with a personal or family history of asthma or allergic rhinitis. Associations include phenylketonuria and certain immunodeficiency states, e.g. Wiskott–Aldrich, ataxia telangiectasia, X-linked agammaglobulinaemia. Dermographism occurs in 1.5–4.2% of the normal population. There is a transient pruritic wheal after the skin is stroked by a firm object. This property can be transferred by the IgE fraction of serum. Cataracts are a serious complication of severe atopic dermatitis, most commonly developing in the second and third decades.

11.3 B, D

Urticaria primarily involves the skin, causing transient, erythematous circumscribed areas of oedema. However, oedema of the gastrointestinal and respiratory tracts may also occur. If the cutaneous oedema involves the deep dermis or subcutaneous tissues, it is called 'angioedema'. Urticaria alone is not a manifestation of heriditary angioedema. More than 20% of the population experience urticaria at some time. In 75% of cases the cause is unknown. Some cases are associated with Type I hypersensitivity, drugs (e.g. penicillin, aspirin, histamine-releasing drugs), malignancies or physical agents (e.g. heat, cold, pressure).

11.4 Which of the following is/are features of the Henoch–Schönlein syndrome?

A. A flexurally distributed, erythematous, maculopapular exanthem.
B. Non-migratory polyarthralgia.
C. Intussusception.
D. Haematuria.
E. A steroid-responsive glomerulonephritis.

11.5 Which of the following is/are true concerning dermatitis herpetiformis?

A. It is invariably associated with a gluten-sensitive enteropathy.
B. It is characterised by the deposition of IgE in the affected skin.
C. It is characterised by the deposition of IgA in normal and perilesional skin.
D. It is eleviated by topical iodine.
E. It is associated with anti-reticulin antibodies.

11.6 Pemphigus is characterised by which of the following?

A. Subepidermal bullae.
B. Serum IgG against the basement membrane of the skin.
C. Deposition of IgG and complement (C3) along the basement membrane.
D. Serum IgG against squamous epithelial intercellular substances.
E. A positive Nikolsky's sign.

Answers overleaf

11.4 B, C, D

This syndrome of young children and adults is often preceded by a history of infection. The underlying lesion is an allergic vasculitis, which manifests itself by palpable purpura on the extensor surfaces of the extremities and buttocks, glomerulonephritis, and polyarthralgia. Abdominal involvement due to oedema and haemorrhage in the small bowel may lead to melaena and sometimes intussusception. Whereas the abdominal and joint involvements are steroid sensitive, the skin and renal lesions are resistant. The long-term prognosis is good, provided chronic renal failure does not develop.

11.5 C, E

Dermatitis herpetiformis is typified by a chronic intensely pruritic bullous exanthem. Up to 81% of cases are associated with coeliac disease but its response to a gluten-free diet is controversial. IgA deposits are found in normal and perilesional skin but not in the active lesions themselves. There are also small deposits of IgG, IgM and complement. Anti-reticulin antibody is an IgG immunoglobulin which cross-reacts with gluten. The lesions are aggravated by halogens such as iodine and eleviated by dapsone.

11.6 D, E

Pemphigus is a potentially fatal disorder in which acantholytic intraepidermal bullae develop in the skin and/or mucous membranes. The epidermis is therefore easily detached from underlying skin (Nikolsky's sign). Diagnosis is possible by the demonstration of antibodies, in the skin and serum, directed against intercellular substances. In contrast, pemphigoid is more benign and characterised by subepidermal bullae which do not rupture so easily; antibody is directed against the basement membrane of the skin, where deposits of IgG and C3 are detectable.

11.7 Which of the following is/are true concerning the lesions of erythema multiforme?

A. They are associated with IgM deposition in and around dermal blood vessels.
B. They are symmetrically distributed and polymorphic in appearance.
C. Most characteristically, they include 'iris' or 'target' lesions.
D. They are not associated with systemic symptoms.
E. They are pruritic.

11.8 With which of the following is erythema nodosum associated?

A. Lymphoma.
B. Sarcoidosis.
C. Streptococcal infections.
D. Ulcerative colitis.
E. Oral contraceptives.

II: Respiratory Medicine

11.9 Pulmonary eosinophilia is associated with which of the following?

A. *Ascaris lumbricoides.*
B. *Strongyloides stercoralis.*
C. *Ancylostoma braziliense.*
D. Nickel carbonyl.
E. Chlorpropamide.

11.10 Concerning sarcoidosis, which of the following is/are true?

A. Histology is characterised by caseating epithelioid granulomas.
B. Hilar lymphadenopathy is always bilateral.
C. Hypergammaglobulinaemia is common in active disease.
D. A positive Kveim test distinguishes sarcoid from all other granulomatous disorders.
E. A tuberculin test is invariably negative.

Answers overleaf

11.7 A, B, C

Erythema multiforme is a polymorphic mucocutaneous disorder associated with IgM deposition in and around dermal blood vessels. The characteristic lesion is one of a concentric red ring with a dark centre like an iris or target. Itching is usually absent. Systemic symptoms include pyrexia, diarrhoea and joint pain. More severe cases (Stevens–Johnson syndrome) may be fatal. Many cases are idiopathic. Others are precipitated by, for example, drugs (e.g. penicillin, sulphonamides) and infections (e.g. mycoplasma, herpes simplex).

11.8 B, C, D, E

Erythema nodosum is characterised by tender red nodules, mainly in the pretibial region. It most frequently occurs in young women, in whom sarcoidosis and streptococcal infection are the commonest causes in this country. It is also associated with ulcerative colitis, a variety of infections (e.g. tuberculosis, leprosy, lymphogranuloma venereum and systemic fungi) and drug reactions (e.g. sulphonamides, iodides and contraceptives). It is considered to be a hypersensitivity vasculitis.

11.9 All true

All the above can produce a condition referred to as Löffler's pneumonia. Pulmonary and often blood eosinophilia is associated with migratory pulmonary infiltrates which are generally peripheral or pleural based. The condition is self-limiting, usually resolving within 1 month. It is thought to be an example of a Type I allergic reaction (see hypersensitivity section). The most notable aetiological agents are the tissue invasive parasites but drugs such as chlorpropamide and para-aminosalicylic acid may be to blame.

11.10 C, D

Non-caseating epithelioid granulomas occur commonly in the mediastinal and peripheral lymph nodes, lungs, liver, eyes and skin. Hilar lymphadenopathy is typically bilateral but occasionally unilateral. Total IgG, IgA and IgM is increased by active disease. The Kveim reaction is positive in 50–85% of cases and the tuberculin negative in about 60%. The Kveim reaction is negative in all other granulomatous disorders. The tuberculin test may be negative in other granulomatous conditions—notably miliary tuberculosis.

11.11 **Which of the following complications of sarcoidosis is/are due to circulating immune complexes?**

A. Bilateral hilar lymphadenopathy.
B. Corneal band opacities.
C. Iritis.
D. Chronic meningitis.
E. Erythema nodosum.

11.12 **Which of the following is/are compatible with cryptogenic fibrosing alveolitis?**

A. Productive cough with copious purulent sputum.
B. Tachypnoea and dyspnoea of insidious onset.
C. Finger clubbing.
D. Antibody against double-stranded DNA.
E. Low titre rheumatoid factor.

11.13 **Caplan's syndrome is characterised by which of the following?**

A. Exposure to coal dust.
B. Arthritis.
C. Circular well-demarcated lesions 5–50 mm in diameter on the chest x-ray.
D. Pulmonary infiltrates restricted to the upper zones of the chest x-ray.
E. Subcutaneous nodules.

III: Renal Medicine

11.14 **A granular or lumpy deposition of immunoglobulins and complement along the basement membrane is seen in which of the following?**

A. Acute post-streptococcal nephritis.
B. Minimal change glomerulonephritis.
C. Membranous glomerulonephritis.
D. Membranoproliferative glomerulonephritis.
E. Goodpasture's syndrome.

Answers overleaf

11.11 A, C, E

Circulating immune complexes are most important in erythema nodosum, polyarthralgia, iritis and bilateral hilar lymphadenopathy. In the last-mentioned, C3 activation products have been found within the first 6 weeks.

11.12 B, C, E

Pulmonary symptoms depend on the extent of pulmonary fibrosis but tachypnoea and dyspnoea are typically present. Occasionally onset is acute and in these cases a cough may be more prominent but sputum is usually minimal. Anorexia, weakness, clubbing and secondary infection or cor pulmonale may occur. The cause(s) of this spectrum of disorders is unknown but may in part be immunological. Antibodies to single-stranded DNA (unlike SLE) and rheumatoid factor are often present.

11.13 A, B, C, E

Caplan's syndrome is the association of large round lung opacities in coal miners with rheumatoid arthritis. Similar syndromes have been described after exposure to silica or asbestos. Histologically the nodules resemble those of rheumatoid lung disease and occur throughout the lung. They usually occur at the same time as active joint disease, subcutaneous nodules and a positive rheumatoid factor but may precede the rheumatoid arthritis. In contrast, 'progressive massive fibrosis' involves mainly the upper lobes of the lung.

11.14 A, C, D

Both immune complexes and anti-kidney antibody have been implicated in glomerulonephritis. In animals, soluble antigen–antibody complexes escape phagocytosis by the reticuloendothelial system and lodge in the glomerular basement membrane where they are seen as granular or lumpy deposits by immunofluorescence. Similar lumpy deposits of immunoglobulins and complement are seen in membranous and post-streptococcal nephritis in humans. In membranoproliferative glomerulonephritis, silver impregnation stains demonstrate deposition on both endothelial and epithelial sides of the basement membrane, producing a 'tramline' effect. In Goodpasture's syndrome anti-basement membrane antibodies are deposited linearly. No detectable deposits occur in minimal change glomerulonephritis.

11.15 **Recognised antigens in human glomerulonephritis include which of the following?**

A. Group A Streptococcus type 12.
B. *Mycobacterium tuberculosis.*
C. Hepatitis B surface antigen.
D. *Plasmodium malariae.*
E. Nucleoprotein.

11.16 **Membranous glomerulonephritis is characterised by which of the following?**

A. Heavy proteinuria.
B. Abrupt deterioration in glomerular filtration rate.
C. Hypertension.
D. Granular casts and erythrocytes in the urine.
E. Hypoalbuminaemia.

11.17 **Minimal change glomerulonephritis is characterised by which of the following?**

A. Lack of specific histological abnormalities.
B. Haematuria.
C. Hypertension.
D. Highly selective proteinuria.
E. Impaired glomerular filtration rate.

Answers overleaf

11.15 A, C, D, E

Mycobacterium leprae, but not *Mycobacterium tuberculosis*, is a recognised cause of immune-complex-mediated glomerulonephritis. Other causes include β-haemolytic group A streptococci (e.g. type 12 and type 4), staphylococci, secondary syphilis, *Plasmodium malariae*, schistosomiasis (bilharzia), hepatitis B surface antigen, systemic lupus erythematosus, anti-tumour antibodies (e.g. bronchial carcinoma) and cryoglobulins. The nephrotic syndrome associated with *Plasmodium malariae* must not be confused with 'Blackwater fever' which may occur in *P. falciparum* malaria. The latter is due to severe intravascular haemolysis, not antigen–antibody complexes.

11.16 A, D, E

Membranous glomerulonephritis is responsible for about 15–20% of adult cases of persistent proteinuria. Proteinuria varies from 5 g to 20 g daily. If sufficiently heavy, the nephrotic syndrome develops with hypoalbuminaemia, hyperlipidaemia and oedema. The urine contains erythrocytes and granular casts (thought to be degenerate cellular casts). Hypertension is not a feature and the rate of progression is slow, with a gradual decline in glomerular filtration rate in most cases. The initiating antigen is generally unknown but a similar histology has been associated with hepatitis B surface antigen and some cases of lupus nephritis.

11.17 A, D

This condition is called 'minimal change' because of the lack of abnormalities histologically. Fluorescent studies fail to show C3, IgG or IgA in the glomeruli. Mediation by lymphocytes is suspected. It accounts for 80–90% of cases of nephrotic syndrome in children and 10% in adults. Highly selective proteinuria is the most characteristic feature. It occurs with oedema, hypoalbuminaemia and sometimes oliguria or hyperlipidaemia. Haematuria and hypertension are not features and the glomerular filtration rate is relatively unimpaired. Remissions can usually be achieved with steroids or cyclophosphamide but relapses are common.

11.18 **Which of the following is/are compatible with a diagnosis of Goodpasture's syndrome?**

   A. Haematuria, rapidly followed by renal failure.
   B. Haemoptysis, preceding the haematuria.
   C. Electron-dense lumps in the capillary basement membrane of the kidney on electron microscopy.
   D. Iron-deficiency anaemia.
   E. High titre of circulating anti-glomerular basement membrane antibody.

11.19 **Berger's nephropathy is characterised by which of the following?**

   A. Haematuria.
   B. Localisation of IgA in the glomerular mesangium.
   C. Increased incidence in Ashkenazi Jews.
   D. An association with heavy cigarette smoking.
   E. Chronic renal failure in the majority of cases.

11.20 **Renal involvement in multiple myeloma may be due to which of the following?**

   A. Hypercalcaemia.
   B. High serum uric acid.
   C. Amyloidosis.
   D. Pyelonephritis.
   E. Tubular obstruction secondary to precipitation of myeloma protein.

Answers overleaf

11.18 A, B, D, E

This rare condition occurs most commonly in young men. The circulating anti-glomerular basement membrane antibody also reacts with the capillary basement membrane of the lung. In the lung a necrotising alveolitis with haemorrhage occurs. In the kidney a diffuse proliferative nephritis develops and immunofluorescence demonstrates a continuous linear deposition of immunoglobulin and fibrin along the glomerular basement membrane. A corresponding granular dense band is seen with electron microscopy. Haemoptysis usually precedes haematuria and the rapid onset of renal failure. A refractory iron-deficiency anaemia develops. Spontaneous regression has occasionally been reported but mortality is very high.

11.19 A, B

Berger's nephropathy is identified by mesangial localisation of IgA, and to a lesser extent IgG or IgM, with C3. These patients are commonly young males and present with microscopic, and intermittently macroscopic, haematuria. There is often a preceding non-streptococcal upper respiratory tract infection. Usually the course is benign but up to 25% of patients develop chronic renal failure. Typically there is a focal proliferative glomerulonephritis. One theory is that following a viral mucosal infection, IgA combines with this antigen to form complexes which localise in the mesangium. It is Buerger's disease (thromboangiitis obliterans) which has an increased incidence in Ashkenazi Jews and typically presents with peripheral vascular ischaemia in young males who are cigarette smokers.

11.20 All true

There are five causes of renal pathology in multiple myeloma. Hypercalcaemia, due to release of calcium from osteolytic deposits, may also occur in other malignancies. Urate nephropathy may follow cytotoxic therapy causing breakdown of cells and nucleoproteins. It can be prevented by allopurinol. Amyloidosis occurs in 5–10% of patients with multiple myeloma. Pyelonephritis is probably secondary to the immunodeficiency which occurs in multiple myeloma. Precipitation of myeloma proteins may be initiated by dehydration prior to an intravenous pyelogram and this should be avoided in multiple myeloma.

11.21 **Which of the following is/are true concerning renal involvement in systemic lupus erythematosus (SLE)?**

  A. It occurs in 10% of patients.
  B. It most commonly takes the form of membranous glomerulonephritis.
  C. 'Wire loop' lesions are pathognomonic of SLE.
  D. It is suggested by a 'telescoped' urinary sediment.
  E. C3 and DNA binding can be used to monitor disease activity.

11.22 **Concerning acute post-streptococcal glomerulonephritis, which of the following is/are true?**

  A. Onset is usually 5 days after a group A streptococcal infection.
  B. The ASO titre must be raised to make the diagnosis.
  C. Immunofluorescence shows continuous linear deposits along the glomerular basement membrane.
  D. Over 85% of cases fully recover.
  E. Haematuria and facial oedema are characteristic clinical features.

11.23 **Renal causes of a low serum complement (C3) include which of the following?**

  A. Membranoproliferative glomerulonephritis.
  B. Membranous glomerulonephritis.
  C. Renal polyarteritis nodosa.
  D. Post-streptococcal nephritis.
  E. Henoch–Schönlein purpura.

Answers overleaf

11.21 D, E

Renal involvement occurs in over 60% of patients with SLE and accounts for more than 50% of deaths. Histology varies but focal is commoner than membranous glomerulonephritis. None of the histological changes is pathognomonic and the classical 'wire loop' lesions can occur in other vasculitidies. They are only seen in advanced cases and consist of localised eosinophilic thickenings of some capillary loops. A 'telescoped' urinary sediment contains more than two types of casts together with erythrocytes and leucocytes and suggests lupus nephritis. Low serum C3 and high DNA-binding capacity suggest an exacerbation.

11.22 D, E

This condition occurs 10–14 days after a streptococcal infection, usually group A type 12 but sometimes types 1, 4, 6, 23 or 49. Streptococci may be grown from the throat and the ASO titre may be raised, but other cases may follow a streptococcal pyoderma and the anti-DNase B or anti-hyaluronidase titres alone may then be raised. Fluorescent studies show lumpy deposits suggesting that soluble immune complexes mediate this condition. At least 85% of cases show full recovery. Chronic disease is more likely to develop in adults. Clinical features include haematuria, facial oedema, oliguria and proteinuria. Complications include pulmonary oedema and hypertensive encephalopathy.

11.23 A, D

Serum complement is normal in renal polyarteritis nodosa, Henoch–Schönlein purpura and membranous glomerulonephritis. It is low in membranoproliferative glomerulonephritis, active lupus nephritis and post-streptococcal nephritis. It can also be low in glomerulonephritis complicating infective endocarditis or an infected ventriculo-atrial shunt. A serum factor (C3 nephritic factor) has been described in patients with membranoproliferative glomerulonephritis which activates the alternative pathway and may be responsible for the low C3.

IV: Liver Medicine

The following three questions compare and contrast primary biliary cirrhosis and hepatitis B surface antigen (HBs Ag)-negative chronic active hepatitis. Please do all three as the answers are given as one table overleaf.

11.24 Primary biliary cirrhosis is characterised by which of the following?

    A. Onset most commonly in young women aged 10–20 years.
    B. Insidious onset, often presenting with pruritus.
    C. Monocytic cell infiltrate with granulomas around the bile ducts.
    D. Association with HLA-B8.
    E. Steroid sensitivity.

11.25 Primary biliary cirrhosis is associated with which of the following?

    A. Rheumatoid arthritis.
    B. Renal tubular acidosis.
    C. Raynaud's phenomenon.
    D. Coombs' positive haemolytic anaemia.
    E. Thyroiditis.

11.26 HBs antigen-negative chronic active hepatitis is characterised by which of the following?

    A. Positive anti-nuclear factor.
    B. Smooth muscle antibody detectable in most patients.
    C. Mitochondrial antibody detectable in most patients.
    D. High serum IgM.
    E. Finger clubbing.

Answers overleaf

11.24 B, C
11.25 A, B, C, E
11.26 A, B

	HBs antigen-negative chronic active hepatitis	Primary biliary cirrhosis
1. Age of onset	10–20 years/ menopause	40–59 years
2. Sex	75% female	90% female
3. Associated diseases	Autoimmune disorders, e.g. pernicious anaemia, Coombs' positive haemolytic anaemia, thyroiditis	(a) Collagen disorders, e.g. rheumatoid arthritis, 'CRST' syndrome (b) Thyroiditis (c) Renal tubular acidosis
4. Common clinical features	Amenorrhoea, spider naevi	Pruitus, clubbing, skin xanthomas
5. Serum immunoglobulins	↑ IgG	↑ IgM
6. Anti-nuclear factor	80%	10–20%
7. Smooth muscle antibody	70%	50%
8. Mitochondrial antibody	30%	over 96%
9. HLA association	HLA-B8 (60%)	None recognised
10. Recognised treatment	Prednisolone, azathioprine	D-penicillamine; cholestyramine (for pruritus); steroids contraindicated (osteoporotic)
11. Liver histology	Lymphocytes and plasma cells in the portal zones and infiltrating between hepatocytes; later fibrosis	Monocytes (mainly lymphocytes) and granulomas around bile ducts; later fibrosis

11.27 **Which of the following is/are true concerning primary sclerosing cholangitis?**

A. Commoner in males than females.
B. Associated with ulcerative colitis.
C. Associated with a raised acid phosphatase.
D. Commoner in the Tropics.
E. Associated with retroperitoneal fibrosis.

11.28 **Chronic persistent hepatitis can be caused by which of the following?**

A. Alcohol.
B. Paracetamol.
C. Ulcerative colitis.
D. Aspirin.
E. Isoniazid.

11.29 **Which of the following liver diseases show(s) an HLA linkage?**

A. Chronic active HBs Ag-negative hepatitis.
B. Chronic active HBs Ag-positive hepatitis.
C. Idiopathic haemachromatosis.
D. Alcoholic liver disease in elderly men.
E. Drug-associated liver disease.

11.30 **Chronic viral hepatitis following hepatitis B (HBV) infection is predisposed by being which of the following?**

A. Male.
B. Very young.
C. South-east Asian.
D. On renal dialysis.
E. A sufferer from Down's syndrome.

Answers overleaf

11.27 A, B, E

In this disease all parts of the biliary tract and gall bladder are involved in a chronic fibrosing inflammatory process typified by an infiltrate of lymphocytes, plasma cell and eosinophils. There is a varying degree of fibrosis leading to presinusoidal cirrhosis. The patient may present with jaundice or asymptomatically with a raised serum alkaline phosphatase. The condition is commoner in males than females (3:1) and associated with retroperitoneal fibrosis, Riedel's thyroiditis and ulcerative colitis. A barium enema is indicated to search for the last-mentioned.

11.28 All true

Chronic persistent hepatitis is a benign non-progressive disease of the liver where the chronic inflammatory cell infiltrate is confined to the portal tracts. The lobular architecture remains intact and there is no piecemeal necrosis of liver cells. Apart from the above, other causes include hepatitis B, non-A non-B hepatitis, Crohn's disease and cytotoxic drugs.

11.29 A, C, D

	HLA linkage
Chronic active HBs Ag-negative hepatitis	A1B8
Idiopathic haemachromatosis	A3B7
Alcoholic liver disease in elderly men	B8
Drug-associated liver disease	None
Chronic active HBs Ag-positive hepatitis	None

11.30 All true

5–10% of patients with HBV infection go on to develop chronic liver disease or the chronic carrier state. Chronicity is more likely in all the above, probably due to an abnormality in the host's immune response.

11.31 Extrahepatic manifestations of hepatitis B (HBV) include which of the following?

    A. Pulmonary fibrosis.
    B. Uveitis.
    C. Hypercalcaemia.
    D. Arthritis.
    E. Hypertension.

V: Endocrine Medicine

11.32 Concerning type 1 (juvenile) diabetes mellitus, which of the following is/are true?

    A. Islet cell antibody is detectable in 40% of cases at the time of diagnosis.
    B. The proportion of cases with islet cell antibodies increases with advancing years.
    C. Diabetes is of gradual onset.
    D. HLA-B8 is the HLA antigen most closely linked to the disease.
    E. Patients invariably need insulin.

11.33 Concerning Graves' disease, which of the following is/are true?

    A. Thyroid-stimulating hormone (TSH) is elevated.
    B. Long-acting thyroid stimulator (LATS) is invariably detectable.
    C. Exophthalmos may be unilateral.
    D. Eye manifestations can occur in euthyroid patients.
    E. Neonates may temporarily suffer from hyperthyroidism due to passage of thyroid-stimulating antibody across the placenta.

Answers overleaf

11.31 D, E

Extrahepatic manifestations of HBV are probably mediated by immune complexes and include arthritis, serum-sickness-like illnesses, vasculitis, cryoglobulinaemia and glomerulonephritis. The vasculitis may resemble polyarteritis nodosa and either this or glomerulonephritis may be responsible for hypertension.

11.32 E

Type 1 (juvenile) diabetes differs from type 2 (maturity onset) in: (1) age of onset (peak at 12 years); (2) acute onset and frequent ketoacidosis; (3) absolute insulin lack so that these patients need insulin; (4) presence of islet cell antibody in 80% of cases at time of diagnosis—the percentage subsequently declines with age but a small minority group (type 2B) remains persistently positive and these patients are more likely to suffer from other autoimmune disorders such as Hashimoto's thyroiditis; (5) HLA association with DW3 and DW4 and, to a lesser extent, HLA-B8.

11.33 C, D, E

In Graves' disease, hyperthyroidism is attributable to the presence of thyroid-stimulating immunoglobulins (TSI) and not to raised TSH levels. TSI mimics the action of TSH and may act via the TSH receptor. Being an IgG antibody, it can cross the placenta and cause neonatal hyperthyroidism. The term LATS is applied to TSI activity detected by a particular mouse bioassay. It is relatively insensitive and not all patients with Graves' disease have LATS. The exact percentages of patients with Graves' disease with detectable TSI vary with the criteria used for diagnosis and the assay technique used. Ophthalmic manifestations are usually bilateral but may be unilateral and are a relatively common cause of unilateral exophthalmos. They can occur in euthyroid patients.

11.34 **Autoantibody directed against the microsomes of thyroid cells is detectable using a haemagglutination technique in which of the following?**

A. 55% of patients with Hashimoto's thyroiditis.
B. 25% of patients with Graves' disease.
C. 10% of adults without thyroid disease.
D. Slightly more often than thyroglobulin antibody in normal subjects.
E. 90% of patients with idiopathic myxoedema.

11.35 **Autoimmune Addison's disease is associated with which of the following?**

A. Vitiligo.
B. Pigmentation.
C. Hypernatraemia.
D. Hashimoto's thyroiditis.
E. Hypokalaemia.

11.36 **Autoantibodies have been found to which of the following receptors?**

A. Luteinizing hormone receptors.
B. Acetylcholine receptors.
C. Follicle-stimulating hormone receptors.
D. Human chorionic gonadotrophin receptors.
E. Insulin receptors.

VI: Haematology

11.37 **Which of the following is/are true concerning a person of blood group O?**

A. He will have serum antibodies to blood group A.
B. He will have serum antibodies to blood group B.
C. He may have a parent of blood group A or B.
D. He is at increased risk of duodenal ulceration.
E. He is at increased risk of carcinoma of the stomach.

Answers overleaf

11.34 C, E

Microsomal antibody is detectable, using a haemagglutination technique, in 95% of cases of Hashimoto's thyroiditis, 90% of patients with idiopathic myxoedema, 55–80% of cases of Graves' disease and about 10% of normal adults. A high titre of thyroglobulin antibody is found in 55% of Hashimoto's and 25% of Graves' disease; 10–20% of normal subjects have detectable thyroglobulin antibody.

11.35 A, B, D

Since the advent of effective anti-tuberculosis treatment, auto-immunity has become the commonest demonstrable cause of Addison's disease. There are antibodies to adrenocortical tissue and associated autoimmune disorders such vitiligo and Hashimoto's thyroiditis. Pigmentation, especially in skin creases and around the teeth, is due to melanocyte stimulation by adrenocorticotrophic hormone, the level of which is high. The plasma cortisol level is low and associated with hyponatraemia and hyperkalaemia.

11.36 B, E

Apart from thyroid-stimulating immunoglobulin, autoantibodies to acetylcholine receptors have been described in myasthenia gravis and autoantibodies to insulin receptors have been described in some cases of insulin-resistant diabetes. Some patients with allergic rhinitis and asthma may have autoantibodies to beta-adrenergic receptors.

11.37 A, B, C, D

Persons of blood group O were once regarded as 'universal donors' because their red cells contain neither A nor B blood group antigens. However, their serum contains antibodies against A and B and sometimes these are potent enough to destroy red cells of A, B or AB recipients. Moreover, transfusion reactions may occur due to the presence of rare blood group antigens. Therefore group O blood should not be used indiscriminately. The ABO blood group is determined by three allelic genes, A, B and O. Genes A and B determine the blood group. The O gene is recessive so a parent of genotype AO or BO reacts as group A or B respectively. If the person derives an O gene from each parent, the genotype will be OO and the blood group O. Duodenal ulceration is associated with Group O. Gastric carcinoma is associated with Group A.

11.38 Haemolysis following a blood-group-incompatible transfusion is indicated by which of the following?

A. Pulmonary oedema.
B. Lumbar pain.
C. Headache.
D. Urticaria.
E. Haemoglobinuria.

11.39 Concerning haemolytic disease of the newborn due to Rhesus (Rh) D incompatibility, which of the following is/are true?

A. It occurs when the father is Rh(D) negative.
B. It is more likely to occur if the fetus is also ABO incompatible.
C. It never occurs in the first baby.
D. It invariably gives a positive Coombs' (direct anti-globulin) test.
E. It can be prevented by giving the mother an injection of anti-D gammaglobulin immediately after delivery.

11.40 'Warm' antibody autoimmune haemolytic anaemia is associated with which of the following?

A. IgM class antibody.
B. *Mycoplasma pneumoniae* infections.
C. Methyldopa.
D. Systemic lupus erythematosus.
E. Anti-I or anti-i autoantibodies.

Answers overleaf

11.38 B, C, E

Blood is considered suitable for transfusion if the ABO and Rhesus D groups are cross-matched. Incompatible blood transfusions may cause haemolysis of the donor's or, occasionally, the recipient's erythrocytes. The latter is due to antibody in the donor's blood. Symptoms vary according to the rate of haemolysis and include pyrexia, intense lumbar pain, headache, dyspnoea and shock. There is evidence of haemolysis, including haemoglobinuria. Pulmonary oedema is a sign of fluid overload. Urticaria, and sometimes asthma or angioneurotic oedema, occur if the patient is allergic to some substance in the donated blood but is not indicative of haemolysis.

11.39 D, E

The most serious cases of haemolytic disease of the newborn occur when father and fetus are Rhesus factor D positive and the mother D negative. However, any blood group incompatibility between mother and fetus can cause haemolytic disease in the latter. If the fetal erythrocytes entering the maternal blood stream are ABO compatible, Rhesus sensitisation is more likely to occur. It is exceptional for haemolytic disease to develop in a first baby but this can occur if the mother has been previously sensitised by transfusion or previous abortion. Maternal sensitisation can be prevented by giving anti-D gammaglobulin. The presence of maternal antibody on fetal erythrocytes gives a positive Coombs' test.

11.40 C, D

This form of haemolytic anaemia is associated with an IgG autoantibody which combines with erythrocytes at 37° C and is usually active against Rhesus antigens c or e. It may be idiopathic or associated with systemic lupus erythematosus, lymphoreticular malignancies or, in children, infections. *Mycoplasma pneumoniae* is associated with 'cold' antibody haemolytic anaemia, due to an anti-I or anti-i IgM autoantibody. The antibodies associate with erythrocytes at lower temperatures and the resulting haemagglutination in the cool extremities may precipitate Raynaud's phenomenon. Methyldopa produces a dose-related reversible haemolytic anaemia due to an IgG antibody with Rhesus specificity.

11.41 **Which of the following is/are true concerning the autoantibody associated with paroxysmal cold haemoglobinuria?**

A. It is an IgM.
B. It combines with erythrocytes in cold conditions.
C. It is responsible for haemoglobinuria after exposure to cold.
D. It is directed against the P blood group.
E. It is associated with a positive VDRL.

11.42 **Haemolysis due to which of the following may be associated with a positive Coombs' test?**

A. Dapsone.
B. Methyldopa.
C. Penicillin.
D. *Clostridium perfringens* septicaemia.
E. An ABO-incompatible blood transfusion.

11.43 **Which of the following is/are cause(s) of antibody-induced thrombocytopenia?**

A. Rubella.
B. Systemic lupus erythematosus.
C. Aspirin.
D. Sedormid.
E. Quinine.

Answers overleaf

11.41 B, C, D, E

This antibody, described by Donath and Landsteiner, differs from other cold agglutinins causing haemolysis in being of IgG class and anti-P. Clinically it is characterised by haemoglobinuria after exposure to cold. Syphilis was said to be the commonest cause of this condition but a positive VDRL must be treated with reserve since false positives are not uncommon in autoimmune haemolytic anaemias.

11.42 B, C, E

The presence of haemolytic antibody coating the red cells can often be detected by an antibody to immunoglobulin. The presence of the haemolytic antibody alone is insufficient to agglutinate the cells in a saline suspension, but when the anti-globulin is added, cross-linking occurs resulting in agglutination. This is the direct anti-globulin or Coombs' test. In the indirect Coombs' test, haemolytic antibodies in the patient's serum are detected by adding the serum to washed erythrocytes and then adding anti-globulin. The Coombs' test may therefore be positive in any form of antibody-induced haemolysis, including cold and warm antibody haemolytic anaemias (as may occur with methyldopa or penicillin), haemolytic disease of the newborn or incompatible blood transfusion. False negatives may occur when there is very little haemolytic antibody present. Dapsone damages red cells by its direct oxidant action. *Clostridium perfringens* probably induces haemolysis via its α-toxin, which is a lecithinase.

11.43 A, B, D, E

Autoimmune thrombocytopenia may be idiopathic ('idiopathic thrombocytopenic purpura') or secondary to systemic lupus erythematosus, especially when it occurs in young women. More acute cases are commoner in young children and often follow an infection such as rubella. The prognosis in these children is very good. In a few individual drugs such as sedormid, quinine and quinidine induce platelet antibodies, probably by acting as a hapten and rendering the platelets antigenic. Aspirin is not a cause of this phenomenon but is contraindicated in cases of thrombocytopenia.

11.44 **Cryoglobulinaemia is associated with which of the following?**

    A. Chronic lymphocytic leukaemia.
    B. Multiple myeloma.
    C. Rheumotoid arthritis.
    D. Heavy chain disease.
    E. Infective endocarditis.

11.45 **Which of the following is/are commoner in Waldenström's macroglobulinaemia than in multiple myeloma?**

    A. Bone pain.
    B. Diffuse lymphadenopathy.
    C. Renal impairment.
    D. Amyloidosis.
    E. The 'hyperviscosity syndrome'.

11.46 **Alpha-chain disease is characterised by which of the following?**

    A. Excessive synthesis of IgA light chains.
    B. Bence-Jones protein in the urine.
    C. Malabsorption.
    D. Malignant lymphoma of the small intestine.
    E. Increased incidence in the Middle East.

Answers overleaf

11.44 A, B, C, E

Cryoglobulins are proteins which precipitate reversibly in the cold and usually consist of IgG or IgM. In otherwise normal people, they cause 'essential' cryoglobulinaemia. Disease associations include multiple myeloma, lymphoreticular malignancies, collagen disorders (e.g. rheumatoid arthritis), and severe chronic infections (e.g. infective endocarditis). Cryoglobulinaemia does not occur in heavy chain disease. Clinical manifestations include retinal vein thrombosis, purpura and Raynaud's phenomenon.

11.45 B, E

In multiple myeloma, malignant proliferation of plasma cells usually occurs in the bone marrow causing skeletal destruction, bone pain, hypercalcaemia and anaemia. The disordered immunoglobulin synthesis is associated with infections, renal impairment and amyloidosis. Waldenström's macroglobulinaemia shares some similar features but the malignant cells resemble lymphocytes rather than plasma cells and proliferate in the lymph nodes, spleen and bone marrow. Lymphadenopathy and hepatosplenomegaly are commoner than in myeloma. Bone pain, amyloidosis and renal impairment are rare. The 'hyperviscosity syndrome' is commoner than in myeloma, probably because of the large size of the IgM molecule secreted by the tumour cells. It may result in retinal vein thrombosis, cerebral thrombosis and peripheral gangrene.

11.46 C, D, E

'Alpha-chain' disease is the commonest of the 'heavy chain' diseases. It is characterised by a monoclonal expansion of IgA secreting B lymphocytes which release incomplete IgA (α) heavy chains. Free α chains are detectable in the urine in some cases but do not show the characteristic behaviour of Bence-Jones protein on heating. The malabsorption is associated with lymphomatous infiltration of the small intestine. Initially there may be some response to oral antibiotics. Later a frankly malignant lymphoma develops. The condition occurs predominantly in the Middle East in Arabs and non-Ashkenazi Jews ('Mediterranean lymphoma').

11.47 **Concerning Bence-Jones protein, which of the following is/are true?**

A. It is present in the urine of about 70% of myeloma patients.
B. It is characterised by precipitating at 37°C and redissolving on boiling.
C. It consists of a combination of kappa and lambda light chains.
D. It gives a positive Albustix test.
E. It is associated with an increased risk of renal failure.

VII: Myasthenia gravis

11.48 **Which of the following is/are true concerning myasthenia gravis?**

A. The defect is presynaptic.
B. Repeated muscle contractions increase muscular strength.
C. There is hyporeflexia.
D. There is an association with oat cell carcinoma of the lung.
E. The disease is also known as the Eaton–Lambert syndrome.

Answers overleaf

11.47 A, E

This protein is present in the urine of about 70% of myeloma patients, especially those with the more undifferentiated type of disease, and is associated with an increased liability to develop renal failure. It precipitates when the urine is heated to 56°C and redissolves on boiling. It is missed by the Albustix test and is only reliably demonstrated by electrophoresis of the urine. It consists of the light chains of immunoglobulin, either pure kappa or pure lambda in type.

11.48 All false

The above all describe a distinct disorder called the Eaton–Lambert (myasthenic) syndrome. The converse is true of myasthenia gravis. Here the muscle shows fatiguability after continued use. Reflexes are normal. Autoantibody to acetylcholine (post-synaptic) receptors is detectable in up to 85% of patients. Myasthenia gravis may be associated with a thymoma. There may be collections of small lymphocytes in muscles (lymphorrhages) and anti-striated muscle antibody is common.

VIII: Amyloidosis

11.49 Secondary amyloidosis is associated with which of the
following?

   A. Tuberculosis.
   B. Hypernephromas.
   C. Rheumatoid arthritis.
   D. Malaria.
   E. Leprosy.

11.50 Which of the following statements concerning amyloid is/are
true?

   A. The major component is a fibrillar protein with a β-pleated
   sheet structure.
   B. In cases associated with multiple myeloma, 'AA' protein is
   present.
   C. The P component is closely related in structure to C-reactive
   protein.
   D. It gives a blue, homogeneous, amorphous deposit with
   haematoxylin and eosin.
   E. It produces green birefringence with Congo red under
   polarised light.

11.51 Amyloidosis is associated with which of the following?

   A. Macroglossia.
   B. Factor X deficiency.
   C. Vitreous opacities.
   D. Vitiligo.
   E. Upper and lower limb peripheral neuropathy.

Answers overleaf

11.49 All true

Secondary amyloidosis is associated with chronic inflammatory conditions such as tuberculosis and osteomyelitis. It occurs in about 5% of patients with rheumatoid arthritis. In developing countries, it is associated with infectious diseases such as leprosy and malaria. Neoplastic disorders are another important cause and include non-lymphoid tumours.

11.50 A, C, E

Each amyloid deposit consists of two components. One, known as the P component, constitutes about 5% and is structurally related to C-reactive protein. It can be seen on electron microscopy to be composed of 10 identical subunits, each with a molecular weight of 22 000 d. The other, major, component constitutes 70–90% of the mass and is composed of 10–15-nm fibrils, in a β-pleated sheet structure. In primary amyloid and that associated with multiple myeloma, the N-terminal sequence is homologous to the variable region of an immunoglobulin light chain (κ or λ). In secondary amyloid, the N-terminal sequence is a non-immunoglobulin protein called 'AA' protein. Amyloid stains pink with haematoxylin and eosin and produces green birefringence with Congo red under polarised light. The latter is the most specific light microscopic stain for amyloid.

11.51 A, B, C, E

The factor X deficiency is due to complexing of factor X with amyloid. Macroglossia is due to infiltration of the tongue by amyloid and infiltration of the spleen leads to the 'sago' spleen. Primary amyloidosis is of three types, the Indiana–Maryland families, the Portuguese–Japanese families, and the Iowa families. They are all inherited as autosomal dominants. Vitreous opacities are found in the Indiana–Maryland families. The Portuguese–Japanese families tend to have lower limb peripheral neuropathies. Iowa families have upper and lower limb neuropathies as well as a nephropathy. Vitiligo is not a feature of any form of amyloid.

12. VACCINES

12.1 Which of the following is/are killed vaccine(s) as presently used?

A. Whooping cough (pertussis).
B. Bacille Calmette–Guérin (BCG).
C. Measles.
D. Rubella.
E. Yellow fever.

12.2 Concerning the Sabin polio vaccine, which of the following is/are true?

A. It is a live attenuated vaccine.
B. It is given subcutaneously.
C. In the UK it is given once during the first year of life.
D. It does not prevent gut infection by wild strains.
E. Most cases of paralytic polio in the USA arise from the vaccine.

12.3 Concerning vaccination against rubella, which of the following is/are true?

A. Arthritis is a common complication in adults.
B. A booster is required after 2 years.
C. Transmission of vaccine strains to contacts is frequent.
D. Vaccine strains can cross the placenta.
E. 20% of young adult females are seronegative in the UK.

Answers overleaf

12.1 A

As a general rule, most viral vaccines are live, exceptions being certain polio, influenza and rabies vaccines. Most bacterial vaccines are in the form of a toxoid (e.g. diphtheria, tetanus), a bacterial polysaccharide (e.g. *Pneumococcus, Meningococcus*) or are dead (e.g. whooping cough, typhoid, cholera). Bacille Calmette–Guérin (BCG) is an exception, being a live non-virulent strain of *M. bovis*.

12.2 A, E

The live attenuated Sabin vaccine has the advantage of being an oral vaccine, which makes it cheap to administer. It also produces IgA-mediated immunity in the gut, which prevents infection by the wild-type virus so that the cycle of transmission is broken. Consequently it confers herd immunity as well as individual immunity. Many live vaccines only need to be given once because they multiply in the host so that the primary immune response merges into the secondary enhanced immune response. This gives high levels of immunity. However, Sabin vaccine contains the three types of polio virus which interfere with each others' replication in the intestine. They may also be inhibited by intercurrent enterovirus infections. Boosters are therefore given during childhood. The main disadvantage of the vaccine is its ability to revert to the wild type in either the recipient or contacts. Most cases of paralytic polio in the USA now come from the vaccine. This is more likely to occur in immunodeficient recipients. In such cases the formalin-inactivated Salk vaccine is safer.

12.3 A, D, E

The aim of rubella vaccination is to prevent transplacental infection and congenital abnormalities in the fetus. 20% of young women are seronegative. The present policy in the UK is to vaccinate schoolgirls aged 11–14 years and seronegative women. In the latter case, it is advised that pregnancy is avoided for 3 months because vaccine strains can cross the placenta. However, the risk of teratogenesis is thought to be low. Transmission of vaccine strains to susceptible contacts has not been observed. The vaccine confers solid immunity for 5–10 years. Mild arthritis is a common side-effect in adults and occasionally occurs in children.

12.4 **Which of the following vaccines is/are associated with neurological complications?**

A. Smallpox.
B. Pertussis.
C. Yellow fever.
D. Rubella.
E. Influenza.

12.5 **Concerning the human diploid cell vaccine for rabies, which of the following is/are true?**

A. It is a live attenuated vaccine.
B. It gives 40% seroconversion after six injections.
C. It should be given after probable exposure to rabies.
D. It should be given prophylactically to people at high risk of exposure to rabies.
E. It is associated with allergic encephalitis in 1 in 2000 cases.

12.6 **Which of the following vaccines is/are contraindicated in the immunocompromised host?**

A. Mumps.
B. Rubella.
C. Bacille Calmette–Guérin (BCG).
D. Pneumovax (pneumococcal capsular polysaccharide vaccine).
E. Salk polio vaccine.

Answers overleaf

12.4 A, B, E

Acute disseminated encephalomyelitis may follow immunisation against smallpox, influenza and rabies. Viral infections, including rubella, may also cause this disorder but it has not been linked to the rubella vaccine. Guillain–Barré syndrome occurred in 354 recipients following vaccination of over 35 million persons with inactivated swine influenza virus in the USA in 1976. In normal children the incidence of persistent brain damage following pertussis vaccination is between 1 in 50 000 and 1 in 100 000. On the other hand, there were 28 deaths from whooping cough in England and Wales from 1977–80, compared to 2 deaths in children who developed a neurological illness within 7 days of immunisation.

12.5 C, D

This inactivated vaccine is the vaccine of choice for humans. It is grown in a human diploid cell line and has very few side-effects so that it is considered safe enough to be given as prophylaxis. Seroconversion approaches 100% and protection appears to be good. Earlier vaccines were grown in brain tissue and were associated with serious side-effects such as allergic encephalitis as well as poorer rates of seroconversion.

12.6 A, B, C

Live vaccines such as vaccinia, measles, rubella, mumps and BCG are contraindicated in the immunodeficient because they can cause overwhelming infections. Additionally, active immunisation may fail to induce an adequate antibody response. For example, pneumococcal polysaccharide vaccines usually elicit good antibody responses in people with untreated Hodgkin's but poor responses in patients who have received chemotherapy and radiotherapy. The inactivated Salk polio vaccine should be used instead of Sabin.

Vaccines

12.7 Specific human immune globulin is available for which of the following?

- **A.** Hepatitis A.
- **B.** Hepatitis B.
- **C.** Rabies.
- **D.** Varicella zoster.
- **E.** Diphtheria.

12.8 According to the British immunisation schedule, a child aged 9 months should have received which of the following?

- **A.** Measles vaccine.
- **B.** BCG vaccine.
- **C.** Smallpox vaccine.
- **D.** Sabin vaccine.
- **E.** The 'triple vaccine' (diphtheria/tetanus/pertussis).

12.9 A young man presents with high fever, pneumonia and a macularpapular petechial rash. It is most marked on the extremities and is accompanied by oedema of the hands and feet. Which of the following is/are helpful diagnostically?

- **A.** A previous history of vaccination with live attenuated measles vaccine.
- **B.** A previous history of vaccination with inactivated measles vaccine.
- **C.** High titres of mumps antibodies.
- **D.** High titres of measles antibodies.
- **E.** High titres of rubella antibodies.

12.10 Concerning adjuvants, which of the following is/are true?

- **A.** They potentiate the immune response to specific related antigens.
- **B.** They accelerate the rate of degradation of the antigen.
- **C.** They activate macrophages.
- **D.** They activate T-suppressor cells.
- **E.** They may be associated with granuloma formation.

Answers overleaf

12.7 B, C, D

'Immune serum globulin' contains antibody from pooled human plasma and is used for the passive immunisation of individuals recently exposed to hepatitis A, rubella and measles. 'Specific immune globulins' are obtained from immunised or recently infected people and are available against hepatitis B, rabies, varicella zoster, mumps and vaccinia. Diphtheria antitoxin is equine, as are antitoxins against botulism and many snake bites. Tetanus antitoxin is now available from human sources.

12.8 D, E

Live measles vaccine should not be given to children below the age of 9 months because it fails to immunise due to the presence of maternal antibodies. Rubella is ineffective in children aged under 2 years. BCG vaccine is given to tuberculin-negative children aged 10–13 years. Vaccination against smallpox is no longer indicated since the highly successful WHO eradication campaign. The triple vaccine and oral polio (Sabin) vaccine are given three times during the first year of life, starting at 3 months of age.

12.9 B, D

The above history is typical of the atypical form of measles occurring in children who have previously received inactivated measles vaccine. Pleural effusions occur and there are extraordinarily high titres of measles antibodies (25 000–200 000 by haemagglutination inhibition test). Mumps and rubella do not produce this picture. The vaccine failed to produce antibodies against the 'F' protein of the virus. This polypeptide is responsible for cell fusion, viral penetration, and haemolysis. Lack of antibodies to the cell fusion factor permitted the measles virus to survive in superficial respiratory mucosal cells by cell-to-cell spread. The other measles virus antigens released by these infected cells stimulated a hyperimmune response to those antigens shared by the inactivated vaccine.

12.10 C, E

Adjuvants potentiate the immune response to unrelated antigens by (1) absorbing the antigen so that it is released slowly for a prolonged period, (2) activating macrophages which then interact with lymphocytes, and (3) activating T-helper lymphocytes and, in some cases (e.g. lipopolysaccharide), B lymphocytes. The activation of inflammatory cells may lead to the formation of granuloma.

12.11 **Concerning complete Freund's adjuvant, which of the following is/are true?**

   A. It consists of a water-in-oil emulsion containing mycobacteria.
   B. The complete adjuvant must be used to obtain any adjuvant activity.
   C. It is widely used in human vaccines.
   D. It is one of the most potent adjuvants known.
   E. Sterile abscesses are a common side-effect.

12.12 **Which of the following is/are adjuvant(s)?**

   A. *Bordetella pertussis*.
   B. Aluminium hydroxide.
   C. Interferon.
   D. Transfer factor.
   E. Bacterial lipopolysaccharide.

12.13 **Which of the following is/are example(s) of active immunisation?**

   A. Subclinical infection by tuberculosis.
   B. Immunisation with diphtheria antitoxin.
   C. Immunisation with pooled human serum against hepatitis A.
   D. Transfer of antibody in breast milk.
   E. Transplacental passage of maternal IgG.

Answers overleaf

12.11 A, D, E

Freund's complete adjuvant consists of killed mycobacteria in a water-in-oil emulsion. It is not suitable for human use because of the intensity of the inflammatory response it evokes and the degree of immunopotentiation. Sterile abscesses may follow the use of Freund's adjuvant. Incomplete Freund's adjuvant differs in lacking mycobacteria and is slightly less inflammatory, while retaining considerable adjuvant activity. Another alternative is to use the muramyl dipeptide component of the mycobacterium, which has adjuvant activity.

12.12 A, B, E

B. pertussis has some adjuvant activity. Aluminium compounds have been used as adjuvants in diphtheria and tetanus toxoid vaccines. Bacterial lipopolysaccharide (LPS) and polyanions such as dextran sulphate are B-cell mitogens. There is as yet no really safe and potent adjuvant for human use. A new approach has been the closure of antigens in synthetic lipid vesicles (liposomes) from which they are slowly released after injection.

12.13 A

Active immunisation may be conferred by vaccination or natural infection, either subclinical or clinical. The remainder are examples of passive immunisation whereby temporary protection to infection is obtained by the administration of preformed antibody. This is achieved by injection of immunoglobulins or by their natural transfer across the placenta or in breast milk from the mother. As this antibody is catabolised or used up by antigen, the protection wanes.

13. PATHOGENESIS OF INFECTIOUS DISEASES

13.1 Which of the following bacterial components inhibit(s) phagocytosis of the organism?

A. The pili of *Neisseria gonorrhoeae*.
B. The M protein of *Streptococcus pyogenes*.
C. The acid-fast cell wall of *Mycobacterium tuberculosis*.
D. The capsule of *Haemophilus influenzae*.
E. The lipid A component of *Salmonella typhi*.

13.2 If a mouse is immunised with a moderate dose of *Mycobacterium tuberculosis* such that it overcomes this first infection, which of the following statements will apply after the infection?

A. It will be immune to subsequent infection by tubercle.
B. It will be immune to subsequent infection by *Listeria monocytogenes*.
C. It will be immune to *Listeria monocytogenes* if this is given concomitantly with tubercle as the second infection.
D. It will be able to transfer resistance to a non-immunised recipient by transfer of macrophages.
E. It will be able to transfer resistance to a non-immunised recipient by transfer of serum.

Answers overleaf

13.1 B, D

The M protein of streptococci inhibits phagocytosis. Variants of M protein form the basis of Griffith typing. The capsules of *Haemophilus influenzae, Neisseria meningitidis* and *Streptococcus pneumoniae* are also anti-phagocytic. Antibodies against these components markedly enhance phagocytosis of these organisms. In contrast, bacteria such as tubercle are not intrinsically anti-phagocytic but continue to grow within the macrophage after phagocytosis. Pili are virulence factors because they enable bacteria to adhere to susceptible surfaces. Lipid A is the toxic component of the endotoxin common to many Gram-negative bacteria. Neither of these last two factors prevents phagocytosis.

13.2 A, C

A mouse immunised with *M. tuberculosis* is protected against challenge by either tubercle alone or tubercle and *L. monocytogenes* given together. It is not protected against *L. monocytogenes* given alone. This is because during the first infection T lymphocytes become specifically sensitised to tubercle. These sensitised cells are rapidly activated when challenged by the same tubercular antigens but not by different listerial antigens. However, these specifically stimulated T cells activate macrophages, which are then capable of killing almost any organism which they have phagocytosed. Hence, non-specific immunity occurs transiently to *L. monocytogenes* if given at the same time as the tubercle. Macrophages and serum cannot be used to transfer specific cellular immunity to a non-immunised recipient since this requires the presence of specifically sensitised T lymphocytes.

13.3 **Which of the following bacteria initiate(s) granulomatous tissue reactions?**

    A. *Brucella abortus.*
    B. *Salmonella typhi.*
    C. *Streptococcus viridans.*
    D. *Treponema pallidum.*
    E. *Mycobacterium tuberculosis.*

13.4 **Which of the following are contained in infectious disease granuloma?**

    A. Macrophages.
    B. Plasma cells.
    C. Epithelioid cells.
    D. Giant cells.
    E. Fibroblasts.

13.5 **Immunological memory, which confers long-lasting protection against a specific organism, is mediated by which of the following?**

    A. Specific T lymphoblasts.
    B. Plasma cells.
    C. Macrophages.
    D. Small lymphocytes.
    E. Langerhans cells.

Answers overleaf

13.3 A, B, D, E

Tissue reactions to non-toxigenic bacteria may be purulent or granulomatous. The former are characterised by a short acute course and early infiltration by polymorphonuclear leucocytes. They are due to extracellular bacteria. Granulomatous reactions are often associated with chronic infections due to facultative intracellular bacteria. Examples include *Mycobacterium* species, *Brucella* species, *Listeria monocytogenes, Yersinia pestis, Salmonella typhi, Salmonella paratyphi, Treponema pallidum* and *Legionella pneumophilia.*

13.4 A, C, D, E

Initially, these granulomas contain lymphocytes and macrophages. Later they contain epithelioid cells, giant cells and fibroblasts. Eosinophils may occur in granulomas induced by parasites. The tightly packed cells forming granuloma reduce the chances of further spread of infection.

13.5 D

The immunity conferred by specific T lymphoblasts (activated T cells) or plasma cells (derived from B cells) is short lived. The life span of these cells is short. Macrophages do not confer specific immunity. Langerhans cells are macrophage-like cells which occur in the epidermis. The 'memory cell' of the immune system is the small lymphocyte which has a relatively long life span (at least several weeks) and confers specific immunity.

Pathogenesis of Infectious Diseases

13.6 Which of the following is/are FALSE concerning humoral immunity against viruses?

A. Antibody can inhibit the adherence of virus to its cellular receptor.
B. Antibody can lyse virus via the classical complement pathway.
C. Antibody can enhance viral pathogenicity.
D. Antibody can prevent cell-to-cell spread of virus.
E. Antibody and complement can enhance phagocytosis.

13.7 'Antigenic variation' is involved in the pathogenesis of which of the following?

A. African sleeping sickness (*Trypanosoma rhodesiense* and *T. gambiense*).
B. Chagas' disease (*Trypanosoma cruzi*).
C. Malaria.
D. Schistosomiasis (bilharzia).
E. Borreliosis (relapsing fever).

13.8 Which of the following is/are thought to be involved in defence against helminths?

A. IgE.
B. IgD.
C. Eosinophils.
D. Mast cells.
E. Antibody-dependent cell-mediated cytotoxicity (ADCC).

13.9 Serum antibody is important in limiting which of the following viral infections?

A. Recurrent rhinovirus infections.
B. Reactivation of herpes simplex.
C. Re-infection with the same strain of influenza virus.
D. Tansplacental spread of rubella virus.
E. The viraemic phase of poliomyelitis.

Answers overleaf

13.6 D

Antibody is particularly important during the viraemic phase of the infection. Specific antibody can neutralise the virus and prevent its adherence to target cell receptors. Together with complement, it can lyse viral particles and enhance phagocytosis. Antibody can also lyse virally infected cells with the aid of complement but it cannot prevent cell-to-cell spread of virus. However, in some circumstances antibody can actually enhance viral pathogenicity. For example, in dengue a haemorrhagic diathesis has been described associated with a second infection by a different strain. This is thought to be due to cross-reacting antibodies which fail to neutralise the second infection.

13.7 A, C, E

Antigenic variation refers to the evasion of the immune response by sequential alteration of surface antigens. Relapses occur each time new antigens occur on the parasite because the host has to redevelop immunity to them. This is thought to play an important part in the pathogenesis of African sleeping sickness, malaria and borreliosis.

13.8 A, C, D, E

IgE-mediated release of histamine and eosinophil chemotactic factor from mast cells may be involved in the defence against helminths. Histamine may have a role to play in the expulsion of intestinal helminths. Eosinophils are known to bind to antibody-coated nematodes and may be the mediators of antibody-dependent cell-mediated cytotoxicity. Helminths are generally too large to be removed by phagocytosis. IgD does not have a role.

13.9 C, D, E

Serum antibody fails to prevent recurrent rhinovirus infections because of the many strains involved and because immunity is largely due to local IgA and not serum IgG. Reactivation of herpes simplex occurs despite adequate serum IgG levels. Transplacental spread of rubella and the viraemic phase of polio are both blood borne and susceptible to serum antibodies. Serum antibody will protect against re-infection with the same strain of influenza virus. However, normally, influenza recurs due to infection with an antigenically different strain to which existing antibody is not neutralising.

13.10 Which of the following micro-organisms multiply inside macrophages?

   A. *Listeria monocytogenes.*
   B. *Streptococcus pneumoniae.*
   C. *Chlamydia trachomatis.*
   D. *Brucella melitensis.*
   E. *Leishmania donovani.*

13.11 Eosinophilia is a feature of infection caused by which of the following parasites?

   A. *Schistosoma mansoni.*
   B. *Taenia saginata.*
   C. *Ascaris lumbricoides.*
   D. *Echinococcus granulosus.*
   E. *Necator americanus.*

13.12 Concerning naturally acquired immunity to malaria, which of the following is/are true?

   A. The primary target is the sporozoite.
   B. The primary target is intrahepatic in *Plasmodium vivax* infection but extrahepatic in *P. falciparum* infection.
   C. The response is purely B-cell mediated.
   D. It is accompanied by hyper-responsiveness to other antigens, e.g. viruses.
   E. It is induced rapidly after the primary infection.

13.13 Which of the following is/are true concerning the delta antigen?

   A. Its incidence is increased in haemophiliacs.
   B. It is associated with hepatitis B infection.
   C. It is a marker of susceptibility to hepatitis B infection.
   D. It is a marker of immunity to hepatitis B infection.
   E. It is a marker of immunity to non-A non-B hepatitis.

Answers overleaf

13.10 A, C, D, E

Many micro-organisms which are ingested by phagocytes can then resist the normal killing process. They multiply within the cell and are protected from antibody, complement and other host defence systems. Such micro-organisms include bacteria (e.g. *Mycobacteria, Listeria, Brucella*), *Rickettsia, Chlamydia,* protozoa (e.g. *Leishmania*), viruses (e.g. measles, lymphocytic choriomeningitis virus) and some fungi.

13.11 A, C, D

Eosinophilia and the production of IgE antibodies are features of invasive metazoal infections such as strongyloidiasis, ascariasis, hydatid cyst disease (*Echinococcus granulosus*), filariasis, schistosomiasis and fascioliasis. Parasites such as hookworms (e.g. *Necator americanus*) and tapeworms (e.g. *Taenia saginata*), which remain in the intestine, do not elicit these responses.

13.12 All false

The sporozoite is only present in the blood for about 30 min after the host has been bitten by the mosquito and thus evades the host's immune system. The immune response, which is both T- and B-cell mediated, is aimed at the extrahepatic stages in all types of malaria. Infected patients tend to be hyporesponsive to other antigens. They develop immunity to malaria only after repeated infections. In the case of *P. falciparum*, this may be due to antigenic variability among strains.

13.13 A, B

The delta antigen is closely associated with hepatitis B infection. It appears to be a transmissible agent dependent on helper function from hepatitis B for its replication. It contains RNA and its predominant form is a 35–37-nm particle. It is commoner in haemophiliacs and drug addicts. In haemophiliacs its presence correlates with chronic active liver disease. It is not a marker of susceptibility or immunity to hepatitis but an infectious agent in its own right.

14. HLA AND DISEASE

14.1 HLA-B8 has been associated with which of the following?

A. Multiple sclerosis.
B. Optic neuritis.
C. Coeliac disease.
D. Dermatitis herpetiformis.
E. Graves' disease.

14.2 HLA-B27 has been associated with which of the following?

A. Post-shigella arthritis.
B. Post-gonorrhoeic arthritis.
C. Idiopathic haemochromatosis.
D. Subacute thyroiditis.
E. Balanitis.

14.3 HLA-B27 has been associated with which of the following?

A. Post-salmonella arthritis.
B. Amyloidosis in rheumatoid arthritis.
C. Uveitis.
D. Juvenile diabetes.
E. Sjøgren's disease.

Answers overleaf

14.1 C, D, E

Other associations include myasthenia gravis, chronic active hepatitis and susceptibility to alcohol in elderly males.

14.2 A, B, E

14.3 A, B, C

HLA-B27 is associated with post-gonorrhoeic, post-salmonella, post-shigella and post-yersinia arthritis. It is also more common in patients with uveitis, balanitis, Reiter's disease, ankylosing spondylitis and amyloidosis in rheumatoid arthritis.

14.4 Which of the following is/are associated with HLA-Dr3?

   A. Chronic active autoimmune hepatitis.
   B. Coeliac disease.
   C. Dermatitis herpetiformis.
   D. Graves' disease.
   E. Myasthenia gravis.

14.5 Which of the following is/are associated with HLA-Dr2?

   A. Ankylosing spondylitis.
   B. Juvenile diabetes.
   C. Amyloidosis.
   D. Optic neuritis.
   E. Goodpasture's syndrome.

14.6 Which of the following is/are associated with HLA-Dr4?

   A. Uveitis
   B. Balanitis
   C. Conjunctivitis
   D. Endocarditis
   E. Idiopathic haemochromatosis.

14.7 Which of the following is/are true?

   A. Idiopathic haemochromatosis is associated with HLA-A3.
   B. Idiopathic haemochromatosis is associated with HLA-B7.
   C. Behçet's disease is associated with HLA-B5.
   D. Cryptogenic fibrosing alveolitis is associated with HLA-B5.
   E. A Japanese patient with HLA-B27 is more likely to develop ankylosing spondylitis than his Caucasian counterpart.

Answers overleaf

14.4 All true

Other associations include juvenile diabetes, idiopathic Addison's disease, and Sjøgren's disease.

14.5 B, D, E

Other associations include multiple sclerosis and tuberculoid leprosy.

14.6 All false

HLA-Dr4 is associated with juvenile diabetes and rheumatoid arthritis.

14.7 A, B, C

Cryptogenic fibrosing alveolitis is associated with HLA-B12. HLA-B27 is associated with an increased risk of developing ankylosing spondylitis in both Caucasians and Japanese. However, the relative risk is far greater in the Caucasian population.

15. SERODIAGNOSIS OF VIRAL INFECTIONS

15.1 Which of the following is/are true concerning the serodiagnosis of viral infections?

A. Serial serum samples should be taken 5 days apart.
B. A falling antibody titre excludes recent infection.
C. A fourfold rise in antibody titre indicates recent infection.
D. Stationary high titres of antibody exclude recent infection.
E. Complement fixation tests (CFT) are the most widely used.

15.2 Concerning the haemagglutination inhibition (HAI) test for viral infections, which of the following is/are true?

A. It is based on the ability of specific antibody to bind to virus and prevent haemagglutination.
B. It can give false negatives due to β-lipoprotein in the patient's serum.
C. It is often strain specific.
D. It is used to diagnose rubella.
E. It is used to diagnose herpes.

15.3 In the complement fixation test (CFT), which of the following is/are true?

A. The complement used is from human serum.
B. The serum being tested must be heat inactivated.
C. Guinea-pig erythrocytes coated with antibody are used as an indicator.
D. Haemolysis indicates positive serology.
E. Excess complement leads to false positives.

Answers overleaf

15.1 C, E

To make a serological diagnosis, two serum samples should be collected, one at the time of presentation and one 7–10 days later. If during this time the specific antibody titre rises by fourfold or more, this confirms recent infection. In some cases a single titre, or two high titres, may be high enough to indicate recent infection. A falling antibody titre indicates that the peak has been missed but does not exclude the possibility of a relatively recent infection since it will depend on how late in the course of infection samples are taken. CFT are the most widely used.

15.2 A, C, D

The HAI test is only useful where the virus possesses the ability to haemagglutinate red blood cells. For example, rubella and influenza viruses can haemagglutinate, whereas herpes cannot. The test is based on the ability of specific viral antibody to prevent haemagglutination. β-lipoprotein is an example of a non-specific inhibitor which mimics antibody and produces false positives. In other words, it binds to virus and prevents haemagglutination. It is thought to be chemically similar to the virus receptor sites on erythrocytes. Inhibition of haemagglutination is often strain specific, so that antibody will only inhibit haemagglutination induced by the specific homologous strain of virus.

15.3 B

Test sera are heat inactivated to remove complement, and then added to antigen with guinea-pig complement (not human). If antibody is present, it combines with the antigen fixing complement. This is indicated by adding antibody-coated sheep erythrocytes (not guinea-pig) which fail to lyse if complement is absent. Hence haemolysis indicates negative serology. Excess complement leads to false negatives.

15.4 A false positive CFT can be due to which of the following?

    A. Bacterial contamination.
    B. Hypergammaglobulinaemia.
    C. The prozone phenomenon.
    D. Anticomplementary antigen.
    E. Egg antibody in the serodiagnosis of psittacosis.

15.5 Which of the following serological markers of hepatitis B virus (HBV) is/are likely to be positive when the patient presents with jaundice 3 months after infection?

    A. Surface antigen (HBsAg).
    B. e antigen (HBeAg).
    C. Antibody to HBsAg.
    D. Antibody to HBeAg.
    E. Antibody to core antigen (HBcAg).

15.6 The HBsAg can be detected in which of the following?

    A. Blood.
    B. Cerebrospinal fluid (CSF).
    C. Semen.
    D. Breast milk.
    E. Amniotic fluid.

15.7 Which of the following is/are true of an HBV carrier?

    A. Infection is nearly always associated with jaundice.
    B. HBsAg is always positive.
    C. HBeAg is always positive.
    D. The level of IgM class of anti-core antibody is high.
    E. The level of IgG class of anti-core antibody is high.

Answers overleaf

15.4 A, B, D, E

The prozone phenomenon occurs where excess antibody leads to inhibition of complement fixation and false negatives. Certain antigens can fix complement in the absence of antibody. Such antigens are said to be 'anticomplementary' and cause false positives. Mycoplasma can behave in this manner. The psittacosis antigen is prepared in eggs, causing false positives if the patient has antibody to eggs. Bacterial contamination and hypergammaglobulinaemia can also give false positives.

15.5 A, B, E

HBsAg and HBeAg both peak with the onset of jaundice, about 3 months after infection. Antibody to HBcAg also becomes positive at this time but the other antibodies do not develop until several months later. Further information is summarised in Fig. 7.

15.6 A, C, D, E

The body fluids listed here are important in that (apart from the CSF) they contain HbsAg and are thus potentially infective. It is worth remembering that the virus does not cross the blood–brain barrier so that CSF is non-infective. However, if it is contaminated by blood during the lumbar puncture, it becomes potentially dangerous. The infective risk is greatly increased if HBeAg is present.

15.7 B, E

The carrier state usually follows anicteric infections. HBsAg is, by definition, positive. The e antigen status is variable. The level of IgM anti-core antibody is low or negative, unlike acute infections in which it is high. The level of IgG anti-core antibody is high.

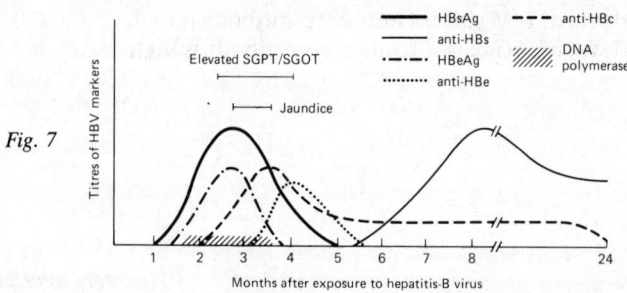

Fig. 7

15.8 Which of the following suggest(s) that an HBV carrier is of high infectivity?

  A. e antigen positive.
  B. HBsAg titre low.
  C. e antibody positive.
  D. DNA polymerase positive.
  E. High titre of anti-core IgM.

15.9 Diagnosis of hepatitis A virus infection in the jaundiced patient is made by which of the following?

  A. Examination of faeces with the electron microscope.
  B. Isolation of virus in tissue culture.
  C. Assay of specific IgM.
  D. Assay of specific IgG.
  E. Liver biopsy and electron microscopic morphology.

15.10 If a pregnant woman comes into contact with rubella at 8 weeks gestation, which of the following is/are true?

  A. The fetus is not at risk if the mother was seropositive before contact.
  B. If seroconvertion occurs, the abnormality risk to the fetus is about 10%
  C. If the patient is seronegative and asymptomatic, no further serology is necessary.
  D. If the patient is seronegative rubella vaccination is advisable immediately.
  E. Infection is usually symptomatic in this age group.

15.11 Which of the following is/are true concerning antibody detected by the Paul–Bunnell test?

  A. It is present in 95% of patients with infectious mononucleosis.
  B. It is able to agglutinate human erythrocytes.
  C. It is similar to antibodies found in serum sickness and some normal individuals.
  D. It is absorbed by guinea-pig kidney cells.
  E. It is of the IgM class.

Answers overleaf

15.8 A, D

	High infectivity carrier	Low infectivity carrier
e antigen	+	−
e antibody	−	+
HBsAg titre	High	Low/moderate
DNA polymerase	+	−
Size of inoculum required to transmit HBV	Small, e.g. needle prick	Large, e.g. blood transfusion

15.9 C, D

Excretion of hepatitis A occurs mainly before the onset of symptoms. It is difficult to detect in the faeces with the electron microscope and difficult to grow in tissue culture. Therefore the diagnosis is made serologically by assaying IgM (single sample) or IgG (serial samples).

15.10 A, E

If the mother is seropositive before contact, her antibody will protect the fetus from the virus. The risk of abnormality in the fetus is high in a woman who becomes infected with rubella for the first time when she is 8 weeks pregnant. If the patient is seronegative, serology should be repeated 4 weeks later to cover the incubation period. Vaccination is inadvisable during pregnancy since its effect on the fetus is uncertain.

15.11 C, E

In 75% of patients with infectious mononucleosis, heterophile IgM antibodies develop with the ability to agglutinate sheep erythrocytes. Similar sheep erythrocyte agglutinins can occur in serum sickness and in some normal individuals. In infectious mononucleosis the heterophile antibody is absorbed by ox erythrocytes but not by guinea-pig kidney. This differentiates it from serum sickness and normal sheep erythrocyte agglutinins and is the basis of the full Paul–Bunnell test.

16. SERODIAGNOSIS OF BACTERIAL INFECTIONS

16.1 Concerning Q fever, which of the following is/are true?

   A. Serodiagnosis is by complement fixation test.
   B. Phase I antigen is prepared by repeated passage in eggs.
   C. Phase II antigen is prepared from fresh isolates of *Coxiella burnetii*.
   D. Patients with pneumonia only react with phase I antigen.
   E. Patients with endocarditis only react with phase II antigen.

16.2 Concerning the Weil–Felix test, which of the following is/are true?

   A. It is based on the sharing of antigens between strains of *Proteus vulgaris* and rickettsiae.
   B. It is positive in all rickettsial infections.
   C. Peak titres occur 1–2 weeks after infection.
   D. False positives occur in relapsing fever, leptospirosis and *Proteus* infections.
   E. If positive, it excludes Brill–Zinsser disease.

Answers overleaf

16.1 A

Phase I antigen is prepared from fresh isolates of *Coxiella burnetii* and reacts with antisera from cases of endocarditis. Phase II antigen is prepared by passage in eggs and reacts with antisera from cases of acute pneumonia and chronic endocarditis.

16.2 A, D

Infection with *Rickettsia prowazekii*, the cause of epidemic (louse-borne) typhus, leads to production of antibodies which cross-react with strains of *Proteus vulgaris*. This is the basis of the Weil–Felix test. Peak titres occur 3–4 weeks after infection. False positives are common and better serological tests are available. Brill–Zinsser disease is a recrudescence of louse-borne typhus and can give a negative or positive Weil–Felix test.

16.3 Which of the following is/are true concerning the anti-streptolysin O (ASO) test?

A. It is specific to group A streptococcal infection (*Streptococcus pyogenes*).
B. It is more often positive after streptococcal throat than streptococcal skin infections.
C. It usually shows rising titres in a severe rheumatic fever recrudescence.
D. When negative, it excludes rheumatic fever.
E. It gives false positives in patients with rheumatoid arthritis.

16.4 Which of the following is/are true concerning a positive DNase B test combined with a negative ASO test?

A. It suggests a group B streptococcal infection.
B. It suggests a group C or G streptococcal infection.
C. It is more typical of streptococcal skin than throat infection.
D. In a case of glomerulonephritis, it suggests prior streptococcal pyoderma.
E. It is a feature of systemic lupus erythematosus.

16.5 The 'quellung test' is used to serotype which of the following?

A. *Corynebacterium diphtheriae*.
B. *Haemophilus influenzae*.
C. *Streptococcus pyogenes*.
D. *Streptococcus pneumoniae*.
E. *Staphylococcus aureus*.

16.6 Which of the following can cause false positives in the *Brucella* standard agglutination test?

A. *Vibrio cholerae* infection.
B. *Yersinia enterocolitica* infection.
C. *Pasteurella tularensis* infection.
D. The prozone phenomenon.
E. The *Brucella* skin test.

Answers overleaf

16.3 B, C, E

A positive ASO can occur in streptococcal group A, C, or G infections. 80% of cases of rheumatic fever give high or rising ASO titres. A negative ASO does not exclude rheumatic fever. It is much more likely to be positive folowing a streptococcal throat than a streptococcal skin infection. 30% of patients with rheumatoid arthritis give high titres.

16.4 C, D

The DNase B test, unlike the ASO test, is usually negative following group C or G streptococcal infections and is therefore relatively specific for group A infections. It is more likely to be positive in streptococcal skin infections than the ASO test and so a positive DNase B and negative ASO test suggest a skin infection rather than a throat infection. Rheumatic fever follows throat infections so that both the ASO and the DNase B tests are usually positive. Glomerulonephritis may follow throat or skin infections. Thus the DNase B test is useful in diagnosing glomerulonephritis following a skin infection as it is more likely to be positive than the ASO test.

16.5 B, D

The quellung test is based on the capsule-swelling phenomenon observed when specific antibody is mixed with bacteria of the homologous serotype. *S. pneumoniae* and *H. influenzae* are both encapsulated and the antigenic structure of the capsule determines the serotype. *S. pneumoniae* type 3 and *H. influenzae* type b are particularly virulent. Before the advent of penicillin, the quellung test was used to serotype *S. pneumoniae* so that type-specific antisera could be used in the treatment of infection.

16.6 A, B, C, E

The most reliable serological screening test for brucellosis is the standard tube agglutination test. This measures antibodies directed predominantly against *Brucella* lipopolysaccharide antigens. A fourfold or greater rise in titre for sera drawn 1–4 weeks apart is indicative of recent exposure to *Brucella* or *Brucella*-like antigens. Such antigens include the *Brucella* skin test, cholera vaccination, or infection with *Vibrio cholerae*, *Pasteurella tularensis* or *Yersinia enterocolitica*. The prozone phenomenon occurs when visible reaction is inhibited by excess antibody, leading to false negatives. Dilution of sera will overcome this.

16.7 **In the serological diagnosis of brucellosis, which of the following is/are true?**

A. A strongly positive standard agglutination test ($> 1:80$) in a symptomatic patient is highly suggestive of acute brucellosis.
B. A positive complement fixation test is strong evidence of continuing infection.
C. Levels of complement fixing antibodies decline rapidly in chronic disease.
D. The standard agglutination test is the most useful in the follow-up of treated cases.
E. Titres must be interpreted in the light of the occupation of the patient.

16.8 **The cause of primary atypical pneumonia can be determined using the complement fixation test for which of the following?**

A. *Chlamydia psittaci.*
B. *Coxiella burnetii.*
C. *Mycoplasma pneumoniae.*
D. *Legionella pneumophila.*
E. Cytomegalovirus.

16.9 **The complement fixation test can be used to diagnose which of the following?**

A. Syphilis.
B. Borreliosis.
C. Leptospirosis.
D. Yaws.
E. Trypanosomiasis.

16.10 **Which of the following tests detect(s) anti-treponemal 'reaginic' antibody?**

A. The *Treponema pallidum* immobilisation test (TPI).
B. The Venereal Disease Reference Laboratory test (VDRL).
C. The Wassermann reaction (WR).
D. The absorbed fluorescent treponemal antibody test (FTA-ABS).
E. The *Treponema pallidum* haemagglutination assay (TPHA).

Answers overleaf

16.7 A, B, E

	Standard agglutination test	Complement fixation test
Detects	IgM and IgG	IgG
In acute cases	+	+
In chronic cases	− or weak +	+
In treated cases	− or weak +	−
	Titres may persist indefinitely	Titres decline rapidly with successful treatment and are therefore useful in follow-up

Positive serology may be due to exposure rather than disease and therefore titres must be interpreted taking into account the patient's occupation.

16.8 A, B, C, E

Legionnaire's disease is diagnosed by the indirect fluorescent antibody test.

16.9 A, C, D

In borreliosis and trypanosomiasis the organisms show antigenic variation so that no suitable antigen has been developed on which to base a complement fixation test.

16.10 B, C

'Reaginic antibody' is formed in syphilis and cross-reacts with a lipid antigen, cardiolipin, which is found in many normal tissues. It is uncertain why patients with syphilis produce this antibody, which was first discovered by Wassermann. The Wassermann reaction has since been replaced by tests such as the VDRL and the rapid plasma reagin test. The antigens used in the other tests are of spirochaetal origin and assay specific treponemal antibody. The term 'reaginic antibody' has also been used to refer to IgE in atopics.

16.11 **Which of the following tests detect(s) mainly IgG anti-treponemal antibody?**

    A. VDRL.
    B. Wassermann reaction (WR).
    C. TPHA.
    D. Rapid plasma reagin (RPR).
    E. TPI.

16.12 **Which of the following is/are true concerning the VDRL test?**

    A. It is a flocculation test.
    B. Once positive, it persists for many years in treated patients.
    C. It is less sensitive than the TPI test in diagnosing primary syphilis.
    D. It is less specific than the TPI test.
    E. It can give false negatives with high titres.

16.13 **Which of the following may give false positives in systemic lupus erythematosus (SLE)?**

    A. VDRL.
    B. FTA-ABS.
    C. TPHA.
    D. WR.
    E. TPI.

16.14 **A positive VDRL with a negative TPHA is compatible with which of the following?**

    A. Treated yaws.
    B. Malaria.
    C. Old age.
    D. Treated syphilis.
    E. Smallpox vaccination.

Answers overleaf

16.11 C, E

TPHA and TPI detect antibody specific to the treponeme, which is of the IgG class. In contrast, the VDRL, WR and RPR detect non-specific reaginic antibody which is mainly of the IgM class.

16.12 A, D, E

The TPI test is more specific than the VDRL but less sensitive in diagnosing primary and secondary syphilis. The VDRL titre falls with successful treatment. False negatives occur at high titres due to the prozone phenomenon. Flocculation is a special kind of precipitation reaction in which cardiolipin (purified diphosphatidyl glycerol) extracted from bovine heart is used as the antigen. Lecithin and cholesterol are added to form a reliable antigen.

16.13 A, B, C, D

Biological false positives for syphilis are noted in about 15% of patients with SLE. They may be the first laboratory clue to the diagnosis of SLE and may precede symptoms by years. The TPI test remains negative in SLE because it is the most specific test for treponemal infection, relying on the ability of antibody to immobilise live *T. pallidum*. However, the TPI test is a difficult and dangerous test to perform and may give false positives due to the presence of antibiotics in normal patient serum. False positive FTA-ABS and TPHA are rarer than a false positive VDRL but occur in about 2% of cases. FTA-ABS may give false positives in SLE and liver disease and TPHA in SLE, skin diseases and pregnancy.

16.14 B, C, E

This combination suggests a biological false positive, which may in part be due to release of lipoidal antigens from damaged tissue. Yaws gives a true positive and, like syphilis, the VDRL becomes negative in treated or burnt-out cases whereas the TPHA remains positive indefinitely.

16.15 A positive VDRL, TPHA and FTA-ABS suggests which of the following?

    A. Untreated early primary syphilis.
    B. Treated early primary syphilis.
    C. Untreated secondary syphilis.
    D. Untreated symptomatic late syphilis.
    E. Treated secondary syphilis.

16.16 A positive TPHA and FTA-ABS with a negative VDRL suggests which of the following?

    A. Treated late primary syphilis.
    B. Tabes.
    C. Burnt-out yaws.
    D. Untreated symptomatic late syphilis.
    E. Untreated early primary syphilis.

16.17 In meningitis, countercurrent immunoelectrophoresis (CIE) of the cerebrospinal fluid can be used to diagnose which of the following?

    A. Tuberculosis
    B. Group B haemolytic streptococci.
    C. *Streptococcus pneumoniae.*
    D. *Haemophilus influenzae.*
    E. *Neisseria meningitidis.*

Answers overleaf

16.15 C, D

For explanation see next question.

16.16 A, B, C

Summary

	VDRL	TPHA	FTA-ABS
Untreated early primary syphilis or false positive FTA	–	–	+
Late primary onwards but tabes usually gives weak or negative VDRL	+	+	+
Early treated syphilis or treated/inactive late yaws or syphilis, including tabes	– or weak +	+	+
Biological false positive	+	–	–

16.17 C, D, E,

CIE is a form of double diffusion performed on an agarose gel, using an electrical potential to promote antigen–antibody interaction, and hence quicken the precipitation. The commonly used antisera in cases of mengitis are:

1. *N. meningitidis* A, B, C, W135 and Y
2. *S. pneumoniae* omniserum
3. *H. influenzae* b.

It is worth remembering that *Esch. coli* cross-reacts with *N. meningitidis* B and *Esch. coli* K100 with *H. influenzae* b.

17. SERODIAGNOSIS OF FUNGAL INFECTIONS

17.1 Serology is useful in which of the following candidal infections?

A. Endocarditis.
B. Vaginitis.
C. Meningitis.
D. Intertrigo.
E. Kidney sepsis.

17.2 Concerning the latex agglutination test for *Cryptococcus neoformans* in the cerebrospinal fluid, which of the following is/are true?

A. It detects capsular antigen.
B. It is positive in 40% of patients with cryptococcal meningitis.
C. It is more sensitive and reliable than direct microscopy of Indian ink preparations.
D. It is more rapid than culture.
E. It is of prognostic value.

17.3 Which of the following is/are true concerning specific antibodies to *Micropolyspora faeni* or *Thermoactinomyces vulgaris* in a patient's serum?

A. They are diagnostic of Farmer's lung.
B. They are rarely present in the acute phase of the disease.
C. They do not cross-react between the two fungi.
D. They are reaginic IgE antibodies.
E. They give high titres after heavy exposure to these fungi.

Answers overleaf

17.1 A, C, E

Serological tests are valueless in superficial or chronic candidal infections. They are useful in deep-seated infections such as endocarditis, meningitis, kidney sepsis and septicaemia. They cannot be evaluated properly without reference to the clinical setting. Alterations in candidal antibody levels tend to be more significant than the presence of antibodies in any single sample of serum. Tests in common use include countercurrent immunoelectrophoresis, whole-cell agglutination and indirect immunofluorescence.

17.2 A, C, D, E

The latex agglutination test uses latex particles coated with rabbit anti-cryptococcal immunoglobulin. Excess cryptococcal capsular antigen in the CSF will agglutinate these particles in more than 70% of patients with proven CNS cryptococcosis. Demonstration of cryptococcal capsular antigen in the CSF is more sensitive and reliable than direct microscopy, and quicker than culture. Loss of antigen from CSF and serum and development of serum antibodies are prognostically favourable.

17.3 C, E

Positive serology indicates exposure and not necessarily disease. High titres indicate heavy or recent exposure. Antibodies are almost always present in the acute phase of the disease but are often absent in the chronic form. They are not reaginic IgE antibodies. The two antibodies are species specific and do not cross-react.

17.4 Concerning aspergillosis serology, which of the following is/are true?

   A. It can be used to differentiate reliably between allergic and invasive aspergillosis.
   B. A diagnosis of invasive aspergillosis is excluded by negative serology.
   C. Aspergillomas usually give high positive titres.
   D. It measures precipitating antibodies.
   E. It is altered by steroid treatment in allergic aspergillosis.

17.5 Rising titres of complement-fixing antibodies suggest dissemination in which of the following?

   A. Histoplasmosis.
   B. Coccidioidomycosis.
   C. Blastomycosis.
   D. Paracoccidioidomycosis.
   E. Mucormycosis.

Answers overleaf

17.4 C, D

Antibodies in aspergillosis are measured by precipitation techniques. Levels tend to be high in aspergillomas and low in allergic aspergillosis. Negative serology may occur in invasive aspergillosis but more often antibody is present in trace amounts (70%). Hence low positive titres are characteristic of both allergic and invasive aspergillosis. Steroids used in the treatment of allergic aspergillosis do not affect the serology.

17.5 B, D

There are no useful serological tests for blastomycosis or mucormycosis. In histoplasmosis, titres do not parallel disease activity. However, in coccidioidomycosis and paracoccidioidomycosis a rising antibody titre does suggest dissemination.

18. SERODIAGNOSIS OF PROTOZOAL INFECTIONS

18.1 Which of the following is/are true concerning individuals infected with *Entamoeba histolytica*?

  A. The latex flocculation test is positive in carriers.
  B. The indirect haemagglutination test is positive in carriers.
  C. The indirect haemagglutination and latex flocculation tests are positive in hepatic amoebiasis.
  D. Intestinal and hepatic forms give similar serology.
  E. The complement fixation test is negative in the carrier state.

18.2 Concerning trypanosomiasis, which of the following is/are true?

  A. A high IgM level in the cerebrospinal fluid suggests sleeping sickness.
  B. Serum serology can differentiate *T. gambiense* from *T. rhodesiense*.
  C. Xenodiagnosis can detect low levels of *T. cruzi*.
  D. *T. cruzi* infection may give a positive Paul–Bunnell reaction.
  E. The serology of *T. cruzi* infection is less sensitive and specific than that of *T. gambiense* or *T. rhodesiense*.

18.3 Concerning leishmaniasis, which of the following is/are true?

  A. The leishmanin test is positive in visceral leishmaniasis.
  B. The leishmanin test is positive in all forms of cutaneous leishmaniasis.
  C. IgG is increased in visceral leishmaniasis.
  D. Serodiagnosis is useful in visceral and cutaneous leishmaniasis.
  E. The diffuse cutaneous 'lupoid' form is characterised by anergy.

Answers overleaf

18.1 B, C, D

	Carrier	Intestinal infection	Hepatic infection
Indirect haemagglutination	+	++	++
CFT	+	++	++
Latex flocculation test	−	++	++
Immunodiffusion	−	++	++

18.2 A, C, D

The serology of sleeping sickness (*T. gambiense* and *T. rhodesiense)* is hampered by the complex antigenic variation which occurs in these organisms. It is impossible to distinguish between the two serologically. They also share antigens with several other protozoa and bacteria. Serology in Chagas' disease *(T. cruzi)* is more specific. Here there is no antigenic variation. Effective complement fixation and indirect immunofluorescence tests are available. Alternatively, 'clean' *Triatomid* bugs are fed on the patient. A 'xenodiagnosis' can then be made by examining these bugs for developing trypanosomes. This is very sensitive. *T. cruzi* can cause a false positive Paul–Bunnell test. A high IgM level in the CSF suggests sleeping sickness.

18.3 C, D, E

The leishmanin (or Montenegro) test consists of a killed suspension of promastigotes injected intradermally. It measures the host's cell-mediated immunity to leishmanial antigens and is thus a measure of host resistance rather than infection. In the disseminated visceral disease, cell-mediated immunity is low and the test negative. It is not always positive in cutaneous leishmaniasis and is negative in the diffuse cutaneous form, which is typically anergic. Serodiagnosis using indirect fluorescent antibody and enzyme-linked immunosorbent assay techniques may be useful, but there are cross-reactions causing false positives, e.g. disseminated tuberculosis, malaria, toxoplasmosis (visceral leishmaniasis) and lepromatous leprosy (cutaneous leishmaniasis). The high serum IgG level leads to a positive formol gel test, where 40% formaldehyde turns the serum into a firm, opaque jelly after 20 min at room temperature.

18.4 Which of the following is/are true concerning the indirect haemagglutination test in cysticercosis?

A. It is more sensitive than precipitation techniques.
B. It yields 17% false positives due to adult worms.
C. It cross-reacts with hydatid antigen.
D. It is positive in *Taenia saginata* infections.
E. It is less sensitive than x-ray changes.

18.5 In *Echinococcus granulosus* infections, which of the following is/are true concerning the indirect haemagglutination test?

A. It gives less than 3% false positives.
B. It is more sensitive than the complement fixation test.
C. It cross-reacts with *Taenia solium*.
D. It is contraindicated by the Casoni test.
E. Titres, after cyst removal, fall more rapidly than with the complement fixation test.

18.6 Concerning the Casoni test, which of the following is/are true?

A. It develops in 20 minutes and disappears in 1 hour.
B. It can be negative in pulmonary hydatidosis.
C. It is likely to be positive if the hydatid cyst has broken.
D. It can give false positive reactions if high antigen concentrations are used in the test.
E. It can be used to diagnose *Echinococcus multilocularis* infection.

18.7 Concerning the serology of toxoplasmosis, which of the following is/are true?

A. The complement fixation test becomes positive later than the Sabin–Feldman dye test.
B. Complement fixing antibodies are usually absent in retinochoroiditis.
C. If the dye test is negative, the patient is unlikely to have toxoplasma retinochoroiditis.
D. The indirect haemagglutination test may be positive for years.
E. The IgM indirect fluorescent antibody test is helpful in diagnosing congenital toxoplasmosis.

Answers overleaf

18.4 A, B, C

Cysticercosis is caused by ingestion of the ova of *Taenia solium*. These hatch into cysticercus larvae which migrate through the stomach wall and encyst throughout the body. X-ray changes of cyst calcification occur after many years. The indirect haemagglutination test is more sensitive than precipitation techniques but yields 17% false positives due to adult worms in the bowel. It cross-reacts with hydatid antigen but is negative in *Taenia saginata* infections.

18.5 A, B, D

The haemagglutination test gives less than 3% false positives. It's sensitivity is 80% compared to 70% for the complement fixation test. However, the complement fixation test's titres fall more rapidly after successful removal of the hydatid cyst. The Casoni test induces haemagglutinating antibodies and therefore should not be performed before blood is taken for serology.

18.6 A, B, C, D

The Casoni test involves injection of *Echinococcus granulosus* cyst fluid and demonstrates a wheal and flare reaction in 20 min if positive. Cyst rupture tends to make it positive. It can be negative in pulmonary hydatidosis. If too high an antigen concentration is used in the test, there can be false positive reactions. Skin tests cannot be prepared for *E. multilocularis* as they contain host protein which will lead to false positives.

18.7 All true

The Sabin–Feldman dye test, the indirect fluorescent antibody test (IFA) and the complement fixation test (CFT) are the three principal serological tests for toxoplasmosis. The dye and IFA are positive before the CFT. High, 1:1024 and above, or rising titres are suggestive of active disease. There is also an indirect haemagglutination test which rises too slowly to be useful clinically and remains positive for years. In toxoplasma retinochoroiditis, the dye and IFA tests are positive in low titre. The CFT is usually negative. The IgM indirect fluorescent antibody test is useful in distinguishing fetal from transferred maternal (IgG) anti-toxoplasma antibody in cases of suspected congenital toxoplasmosis.

19. GRAFT AND TUMOUR IMMUNOLOGY

19.1 A 'tumour-associated antigen' present on the skin tumour cells of a mouse is also likely to be found on the skin tumour induced by which of the following?

A. A different chemical carcinogen in mice of the same strain.
B. The same chemical carcinogen in mice of different strains.
C. The same chemical carcinogen in mice of the same strain.
D. A different oncogenic virus in mice of the same strain.
E. The same oncogenic virus in mice of different strains.

19.2 Which of the following is/are oncofetal antigen(s)?

A. Alpha-fetoprotein.
B. C-reactive protein.
C. Protein A.
D. Carcinoembryonic antigen.
E. Properdin.

19.3 A raised alpha-fetoprotein is associated with which of the following?

A. Primary liver cancer.
B. Secondary liver cancer.
C. Viral hepatitis.
D. Testicular teratocarcinoma.
E. Testicular seminoma.

Answers overleaf

19.1 E

Tumours induced by chemical carcinogens usually have individually distinctive ('private') tumour-specific antigens. Even tumours arising from the same histological cell type elicited by the same chemical in the same mouse strain vary antigenically. In contrast, a particular oncogenic virus will induce tumours in different strains of mice of different histological types which all share the same ('public') tumour-specific antigen. This antigen may or may not be found in the virus. It is specified by the viral genome.

19.2 A, D

Oncofetal antigens are substances which are normally produced in the course of fetal development but are greatly reduced or absent in adults. In certain cancers, dedifferentiation of cells appears to be associated with derepression of the genes coding for these substances and they appear again in the serum or in the tumour itself. They have therefore been used as tumour markers, as an aid to both diagnosis and follow-up of treated cases. C-reactive protein, so-named because it precipitates with pneumococcal cell-wall polysaccharide, is a serum marker of inflammation or infection. It rises earlier (in hours) than the erythrocyte sedimentation rate (ESR) and falls faster with recovery. It is only minimally raised in uncomplicated systemic lupus erythematosus but rises in the presence of infection. Protein A is a component of the cell wall of staphylococci. Properdin is a normal serum protein which activates the alternate complement pathway.

19.3 A, C, D

Alpha-fetoprotein is associated with primary liver cancer (30–95% of patients) and embryonic tumours of the ovary and testis, such as testicular teratocarcinoma (75% positive). It is not a marker of liver metastases or testicular seminoma. Rarely, it is associated with cancer of the stomach or pancreas. Benign forms of liver disease, such as viral hepatitis, may raise levels but not usually as high as in malignant disease.

Graft and Tumour Immunology

19.4 Alpha-fetoprotein is more likely to be positive in which of the following?

A. In English than Bantu patients with hepatocellular carcinoma.
B. In the more undifferentiated hepatocellular carcinoma.
C. If measured by gel immunodiffusion rather than radio-immunoassay.
D. In a child with Wiskott–Aldridge syndrome than one with ataxia telangiectasia.
E. In a fetus with spina bifida compared to a normal fetus.

19.5 Which of the following is/are true concerning carcinoembryonic antigen?

A. It is specific for colorectal malignancy in adults.
B. It is more likely to be positive in metastatic than localised colonic carcinoma.
C. It is more likely to be positive in poorly differentiated tumours.
D. It is negative in uncomplicated ulcerative colitis and Crohn's disease.
E. It is of greatest value in screening for colorectal cancers.

19.6 Which of the following is/are true concerning donor–recipient matching for renal transplantation?

A. Failure of a graft from an identical twin is never due to HLA-mismatch.
B. A graft from a sibling is always preferable to a cadaveric kidney.
C. ABO erythrocyte compatibility is essential.
D. Matching of HLA-Dr is less important than that of HLA-A or HLA-B.
E. A potential donor is contraindicated if the recipient has pre-existing antibodies to the donor's HLA antigens.

Answers overleaf

183

19.4 B, E

There are geographic differences in the incidence of positivity in patients with primary liver cancer. The incidence is greater in regions where it is endemic, as among the Bantu of South Africa (78%), compared to the United Kingdom (30%) where it is much less common. It is also more likely to be positive if the tumour is large, rapidly growing and undifferentiated. If successfully resected, levels fall. High alpha-fetoprotein levels are also associated with ataxia telangiectasia and neural tube defects. Radio-immunoassay is a more sensitive means of measuring alpha-fetoprotein than immuno-diffusion but becomes less specific if low levels are taken as indicative of primary liver cancer.

19.5 B

Carcinoembryonic antigen is not specific for colorectal cancer. It is found in other mucus-secreting endodermal tumours both of gastrointestinal and lung origin. Several non-malignant conditions such as alcoholic cirrhosis, pancreatitis, inflammatory bowel disease and also cigarette smoking can give a positive result. It is positive in 60–95% of patients with colonic cancer. It is most likely to be positive if (a) the disease is advanced, (b) the tumour is not anaplastic, or (c) hepatic metastases are present. Its lack of sensitivity and specificity makes it more useful for follow-up of known treated cases than for screening of undiagnosed colorectal cancer.

19.6 A, C, E

An identical twin is an ideal donor because both major (HLA) and minor histocompatibility antigens are shared. Graft survival from HLA-matched siblings is better than with an HLA-matched non-sibling cadaveric kidney because compatibility in the sibling for HLA-A and HLA-B usually reflects compatibility for the entire HLA chromosomal area. However, if a sibling has neither HLA chromosome in common, transplantation is contraindicated. HLA-Dr antigen matching is more important than that for HLA-A and HLA-B. Pre-existing antibodies to HLA types may arise in recipients following previous organ grafts, blood transfusions or pregnancies and contraindicate transplantation from donors of these HLA types. ABO incompatibility usually leads to hyperacute rejection.

19.7 Which of the following is/are true concerning hyperacute rejection of a renal transplant?

A. It occurs within 48 hours of transplantation.
B. It is mediated by T lymphocytes.
C. It usually responds to treatment.
D. It is associated with polymorphonuclear infiltration of the kidney followed by extensive thrombosis and massive interstitial haemorrhage.
E. It is precipitated by Rhesus antigen incompatibility.

19.8 Which of the following patients is/are LESS likely to tolerate transplantation well?

A. Patients over the age of 50.
B. Patients with diabetes mellitus.
C. Patients who have already rejected a cadaveric kidney.
D. Patients with polyarteritis nodosum.
E. Patients with polycystic disease.

19.9 Which of the following is/are true concerning anti-lymphocyte globulin (ALG)?

A. It is prepared in man by immunisation with lymphocytes.
B. It selectively depresses humoral immunity.
C. It is given intramuscularly in the first few weeks or months following transplantation.
D. It reduces the dose of prednisolone required to produce adequate immunosuppression.
E. It may precipitate anaphylactic reactions.

Answers overleaf

19.7 A, D

Some 25–30% of cadaveric grafts are lost from rejection during the first 3 months. Rejection may be classified into hyperacute (within 48 hours), accelerated (2–5 days), acute (usually within 3 months) or chronic (after 3 months). Hyperacute rejection is mediated by pre-existing antibodies against donor HLA-A, B or C antigens or due to ABO incompatibility. The former may arise following pregnancy or a previous incompatible blood transfusion or graft. Rhesus antigen incompatibility is not important. Treatment is of no avail. Histologically the kidney shows intense polymorphonuclear infiltration followed by thrombosis of small arterioles and glomerular capillaries and interstitial haemorrhage.

19.8 A, B, C, D

Patients undergoing transplants over the age of 50 do less well than younger patients. Diabetic patients have much worse graft and patient survival rates than non-diabetics. This is especially true for those with cardiac involvement and those receiving cadaveric transplants. Otherwise the original disease does not tend to influence the outcome of a graft, although it may recur, as in some cases of glomerulonephritis. Patients with severe multisystem diseases, such as polyarteritis nodosum, derive little benefit from transplantation due to the poor prognosis of the underlying disease. A second cadaveric graft following the loss of a first one does less well, especially if the graft was rejected during the first 3 months. However, the survival of a cadaveric graft following loss of a live related graft is similar to that of first cadaveric grafts.

19.9 D, E

ALG is prepared in horses by immunisation with human lymphocytes. It primarily depresses cellular immunity and it may have some benefit in suppressing acute rejection which is mediated, at least in part, by T lymphocytes. Its main advantage is that it can be combined with lower doses of prednisolone without prejudicing graft survival, and so reduces the side-effects of steroids. It must be used intravenously because it is painful intramuscularly. Disadvantages include increased incidences of herpes simplex infections, anaphylaxis and thrombocytopenia. It is expensive.

Graft and Tumour Immunology

19.10 Which of the following is/are true concerning cyclosporin A?

 A. It is a bacterial metabolite.
 B. It is nephrotoxic.
 C. Ketoconazole is contraindicated in patients on cyclosporin A.
 D. It is a cause of aplastic anaemia.
 E. It is immunosuppressive because it activates suppressor T cells.

19.11 Which of the following is/are true concerning organ transplantation?

 A. Renal transplant rejection is characterised clinically by fever, swelling of the kidney and polyuria.
 B. HLA typing is unimportant for corneal grafting because the cornea is a 'privileged site'.
 C. Rejection is the commonest cause of failure of liver transplants.
 D. Early rejection of a cardiac transplant often presents as an arrhythmia.
 E. Cardiac transplants are predisposed to the development of arteriosclerosis in the coronary vessels.

19.12 Which of the following is/are feature(s) of graft-versus-host (GVH) disease?

 A. An erythematous maculopapular rash following bone marrow transplantation.
 B. Diarrhoea.
 C. Lymphadenopathy and hepatosplenomegaly.
 D. Coombs' positive haemolytic anaemia.
 E. It is mediated by monocytes.

Answers overleaf

Graft and Tumour Immunology

19.10 B, C

Cyclosporin A is a fungal metabolite, used to induce immunosuppression in organ graft recipients. It is not cytotoxic and appears to
act by suppressing helper T cells and on some subpopulations of B
cells. T-suppressor cells and cytotoxic cells are relatively unaffected.
It has little, if any, marrow toxicity and its main side-effect is
nephrotoxicity, which is dose related. Ketoconazole interacts with
cyclosporin A to cause increased plasma levels of cyclosporin.

19.11 D, E

Renal transplant rejection is diagnosed primarily on the basis of fever,
swelling of the kidney, oliguria and worsening renal function. Cornea
(and cartilage) grafts are relatively avascular and well tolerated,
presumably because lymphocytes cannot reach them, but matching
for HLA still correlates well with graft survival. The liver is also a
relatively privileged site and the major causes of loss of liver function
after transplantation are hepatic ischaemia and biliary obstruction
and not rejection. Relatively minor damage following early rejection
of a cardiac transplant may lead to a fatal arrhythmia. The main long-
term problem is the development of arteriosclerosis in the
transplanted heart.

19.12 A, B, C, D

If immunocompetent lymphocytes are transferred to an HLA-
mismatched recipient who is incapable of rejecting them, the grafted
cells will survive, recognise foreign histocompatibility antigens and
react against them. This precipitates the reverse to transplant
rejection, namely graft-versus-host disease. The skin and gut are
commonly involved and there may be lymphadenopathy and
hepatosplenomegaly. Autoantibodies may develop leading to, for
example, Coombs' positive haemolytic anaemia. The rash is usually
the first clinical feature but rarely appears earlier than 5 days after
giving incompatible cells. The danger of GVH disease is related to the
severity of the recipient's immunosuppression and the number of
foreign lymphocytes given. It has occurred in infants with severe
combined immunodeficiency after receiving 50 ml of whole blood.
Lymphocytes, not monocytes, mediate the reaction.

Bibliography

General references

Bier O. G., da Silva W. D., Götze D. and Mota I. (1981). *Fundamentals of Immunology*. New York: Springer-Verlag.
Lachmann P. J. and Peters D. K. (1982). *Clinical Aspects of Immunology*, 4th edn. London: Blackwell Scientific.
McConnell, I., Munro A and Waldmann H. (1981). *The Immune System: a Course on the Molecular and Cellular Basis of Immunity*, 2nd edn. London: Blackwell Scientific.
Roitt I. M. (1984). *Essential Immunology*, 5th edn. London: Blackwell Scientific.

Specific references

Basic immunology

Chapter 1
1.12–1.17
Hudson L. and Hay F. C. (1979). In *Practical Immunology*, 2nd edn, p. 107. London: Blackwell Scientific.

1.19
Halliday W. J. (1971). *Glossary of Immunological Terms*. London: Butterworths.

Chapter 2
Staines N. A. and Lew A. M. (1980). Whither monoclonal antibodies? *Immunology*; **40**:287.

Chapter 3
Lachmann P. J. (1982). Complement. In *Aspects of Immunology*, 4th edn. (Lachmann P. J. and Peters K., eds.) pp. 18–49. London: Blackwell Scientific.

Chapter 4
Howie S. and McBride W. H. (1982). Cellular interactions in thymus-dependent antibody responses. *Immunology Today*; **3**:273.

Bibliography

Chapter 5
5.1
Friedman R. M., Epstein L. B. and Merigan T. C. (1982). Interferon redux. *Nature*; **296**:704.
Mogensen K. E., Daubas P. H., Gresser I., Sereni D. and Varet B. (1981). Patients with circulating antibodies to α-interferon. *Lancet*; **ii**:1228.

5.4
Epstein L. B. (1982). Interferon γ: success, structure and speculation. *Nature*; **295**:453.

5.6
Editorial (1983). 'Toxicity' of interferon. *Lancet*; **i**:1256.

5.7
Editorial (1981). Is interferon any good for cancer? *Lancet*; **i**:1037.
Merigan T. C. (1983). Human interferon as a therapeutic agent—current status. *New England Journal of Medicine*: **308**:1530.

Chapter 6
Owen M. J. and Crumpton M. J. (1980). Biochemistry of major human histocompatibility antigens. *Immunology Today*; **1**:117

6.12
Halliday W. J. (1971). *Glossary of Immunological Terms*. London: Butterworths.

Chapter 7
Turk J. L. (1978). *Immunology in Clinical Medicine*, 3rd edn. London: Heinemann.
Wyngaarden J. B. and Smith L. H. (1982). *Cecil Textbook of Medicine*, 16th edn. Philadelphia: W. B. Saunders.

7.14–7.15
Bell D. R. (1981). In *Lecture Notes on Tropical Medicine*, p. 269. London: Blackwell Scientific.

Clinical immunology

Chapter 8
Purtilo D. T., Yang J. P. S., Cassel C. K., Harper K., Stephenson S. R., Landy B. H. and Vawter G. F. (1975). X-linked recessive progressive combined variable immunodeficiency (Duncan's syndrome). *Lancet*; **i**:935.

Chapter 9
Rubin R. H. and Young L. S. (1981). *Clinical Approach to Infection in the Compromised Host*. New York: Plenum.
Warnock D. W. and Richardson M. D. (1982). *Fungal Infection in the Compromised Patient*. New York: Wiley.

Bibliography

9.19–9.23
Groopman J. E. and Gottlieb M. S. (1983). AIDS: the widening gyre. *Nature*: **303**:575.
Waterson A. P. (1983). Acquired immune deficiency syndrome. *British Medical Journal*; **286**:743.

Chapter 10
Hughes G. R. V. (1979). *Connective Tissue Diseases*, 2nd edn. London: Blackwell Scientific.

Chapter 11
Wyngaarden J. B. and Smith L. H. (1982). *Cecil Textbook of Medicine*, 16th edn. Philadelphia: W. B. Saunders.

Renal medicine
Gabriel R. (1978). *Postgraduate Nephrology*, 3rd edn. London: Butterworths.

Liver medicine
Sherlock S. (1981). *Diseases of the Liver and Biliary System*, 6th edn. London: Blackwell Scientific.

Endocrine medicine
Strakosch C. R., Wenzel B. E., Row V. V. and Volpé R. (1982). Immunology of autoimmune thyroid diseases. *New England Journal of Medicine*; **307**:1499

Haematology
Thompson R. B. (1984). *A Short Textbook of Haematology*, 6th edn. London: Pitman Medical.

Amyloidosis.
Andrade C., Araki S., Block W. D., Cohen A. S., Jackson C. E., Kuroiwa Y., McKusick V. A., Nissim J., Sohar E. and Van Allen M. W. (1970). Hereditary amyloidosis. *Rheumatology*; **13**:902.

Chapter 12
12.2
Editorial (1983). Poliovaccine. *Lancet*: **i**:1022.
Editorial (1982). The relation between acute persisting spinal paralysis and poliomyelitis vaccine—results of a ten-year enquiry. *Bulletin of the World Health Organisation*; **60**(2):231.

12.3
Preblud S. R., Stetler H. C., Frank J. A. Jr., Greaves W. L., Hinman A. R. and Herrmann K. L. (1981). Fetal risk associated with rubella vaccine. *Journal of the American Medical Association*; **246**:1413.

Bibliography

12.5
Turner G. S., Nicholson K. G., Tyrrell D. A. J. and Aoki F. Y. (1982). Evaluation of a human diploid cell strain rabies vaccine: final report of a three-year study of pre-exposure immunisation. *Journal of Hygiene, Cambridge*; **89**:101

12.9
Martin D. B., Weiner L. B., Nieburg P. I. and Blair D. C. (1979). Atypical measles in adolescents and young adults. *Annals of Internal Medicine*; **90**:877.

Chapter 13
13.8
Cohen S. and Warren K. S. (eds.) (1982). *Immunology of Parasitic Infections*, 2nd edn. London: Blackwell Scientific.

13.12
Editorial (1983). Prospects for a malaria sporozoite vaccine. *Lancet*; **i**:1368.

13.13
Editorial (1982). Delta agent, a virus in disguise? *Lancet*; **i**:259.

Chapter 14
14.1
Burnie J. P. (1980). A possible immunological mechanism for the pathogenesis of dermatitis herpetiformis with reference to coeliac disease. *Clinical and Experimental Dermatology*; **5**:451.

14.4
Götze D. (ed.) (1977). *The Major Histocompatibility System in Man and Animals*. New York: Springer-Verlag.

Chapter 15
Grist N. R., Bell E. J., Follett E. A. C. and Urquhart G. E. D. (1979). *Diagnostic Methods in Clinical Virology*, 3rd edn. London: Blackwell Scientific.

15.6
Waterson A. P. (ed.) (1983). *Recent Advances in Clinical Virology*, Number 3. Edinburgh: Churchill Livingstone.

15.10
Miller E., Cradock-Watson J. E. and Pollock T. W. (1982). Consequences of confirmed maternal rubella at successive stages of pregnancy. *Lancet*; **ii**:784.

Chapter 16
16.1
Geddes A. M. (1983). Q fever. *British Medical Journal*; **287**:927.

Bibliography

16.6–16.7
Robertson L., Farrell I. D., Hinchliffe P. M. and Quaife R. A. (1980). *PHLS Monograph Series: Benchbook on Brucella.* London: HMSO.

16.10–16.16
O'Neill P. (1976). A new look at the serology of treponemal disease. *British Journal of Venereal Disease;* **52**:296.

Chapter 17
Mackenzie D. W. R., Proctor A. G. J. and Philpot C. M. (1980). *PHLS Monograph Series: Basic Serodiagnostic Methods for Diseases Caused by Fungi and Actinomycetes.* London: HMSO.

Chapter 18
Cohen S. and Warren K. S. (eds.) (1982). *Immunology of Parasitic Infections*, 2nd edn. London: Blackwell Scientific.

Chapter 19
19.3–19.4
Sherlock S. (1981). *Diseases of the Liver and Biliary System*, 6th edn. London: Blackwell Scientific.

19.6–19.9
Gabriel R. (1978). *Postgraduate Nephrology*, 3rd edn. London: Butterworths.

19.10
Editorial (1983). Cyclosporin and neoplasia. *Lancet*: **i**:1083.

Notes